NEEDLES IN A HAYSTACK:
The Story of Cancer

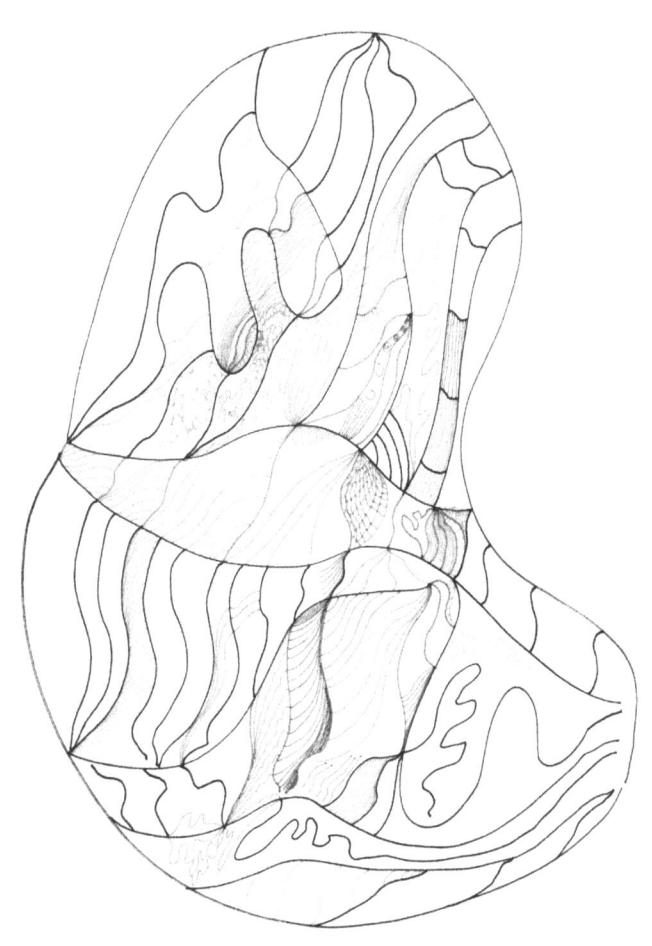

Camilia MacPherson, Ph.D., D.Th.
2016

INTRODUCTION

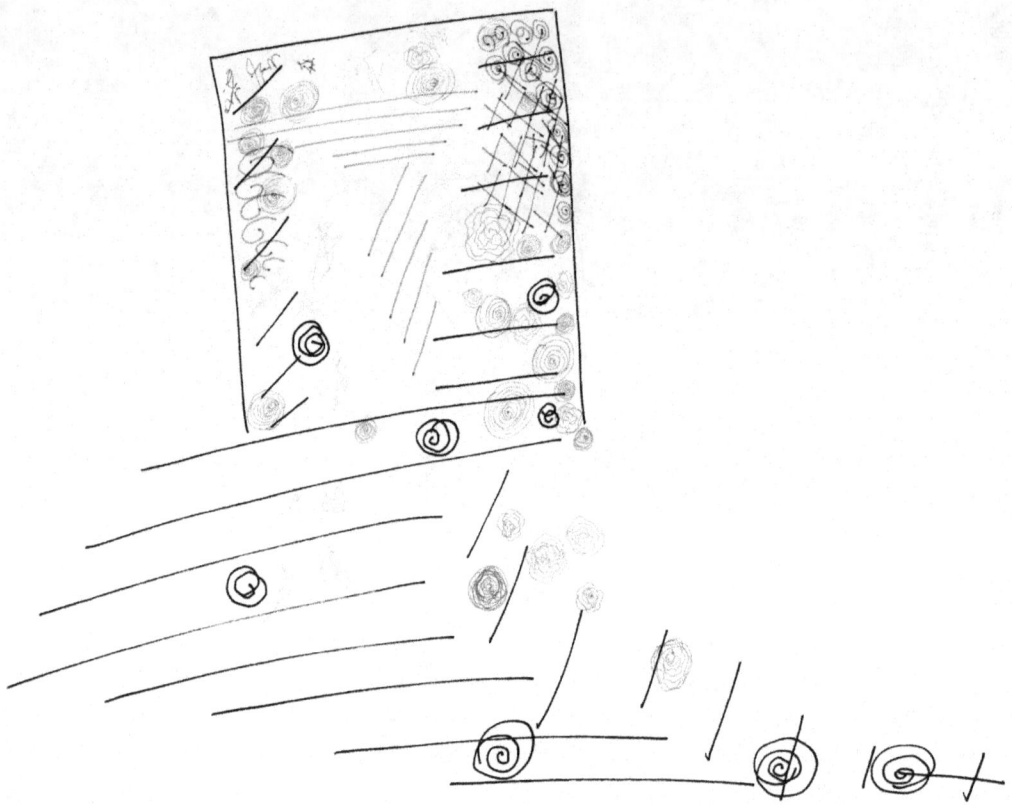

Needles in a Haystack builds on the previous
Volumes 1 to 7 entitled The Story of Cancer.
Automatic Drawings and Surreal
Art are employed in the writing of this book.
It is written in the style of Scholars' Art.
There is no top or bottom of the page, which
contains multiple images. Each page has to be
viewed from every angle and varying depths.

The pre-calligraphy graphics
used in this
book

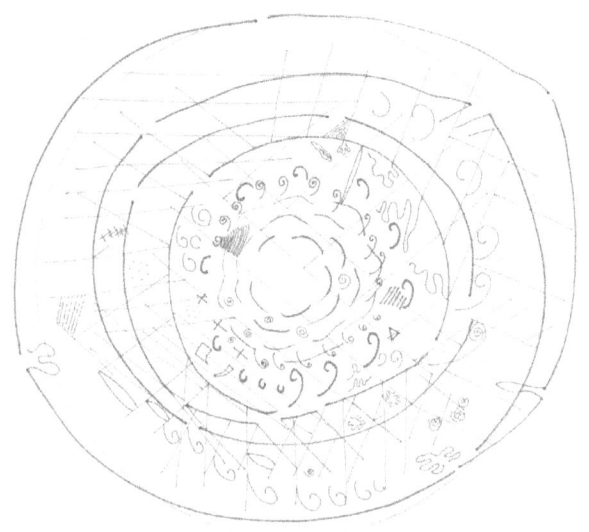

ISBN-13:978-1530587681
ISBN-10:1530587689
Email: tamaracpublishers@icloud.com

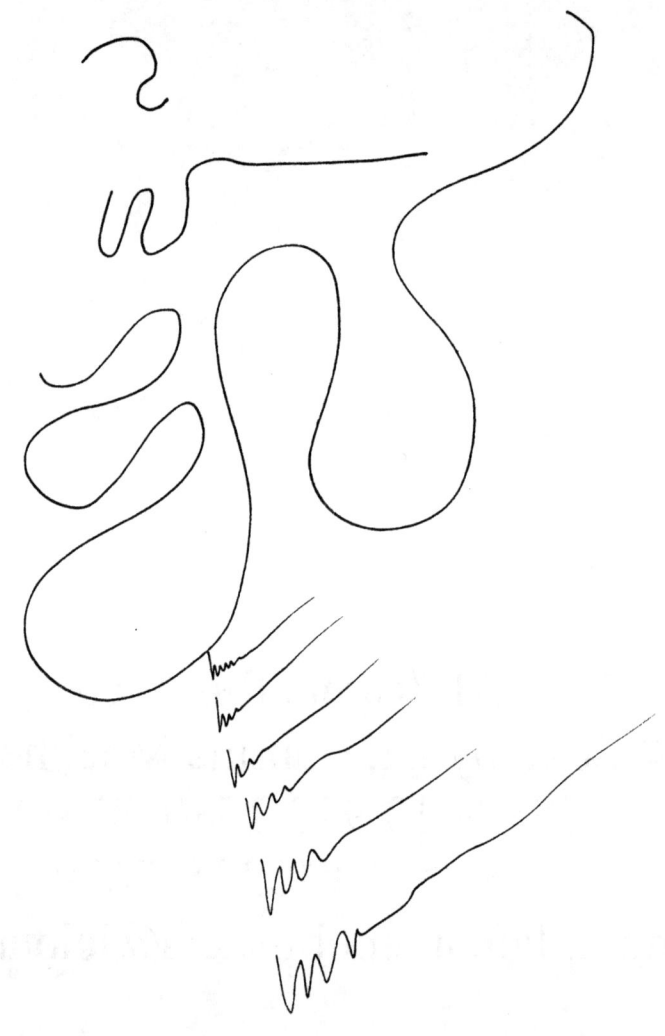

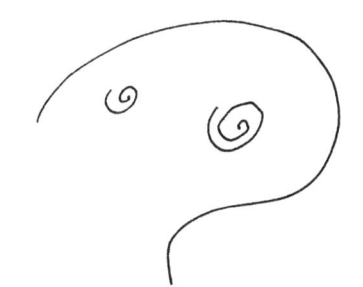

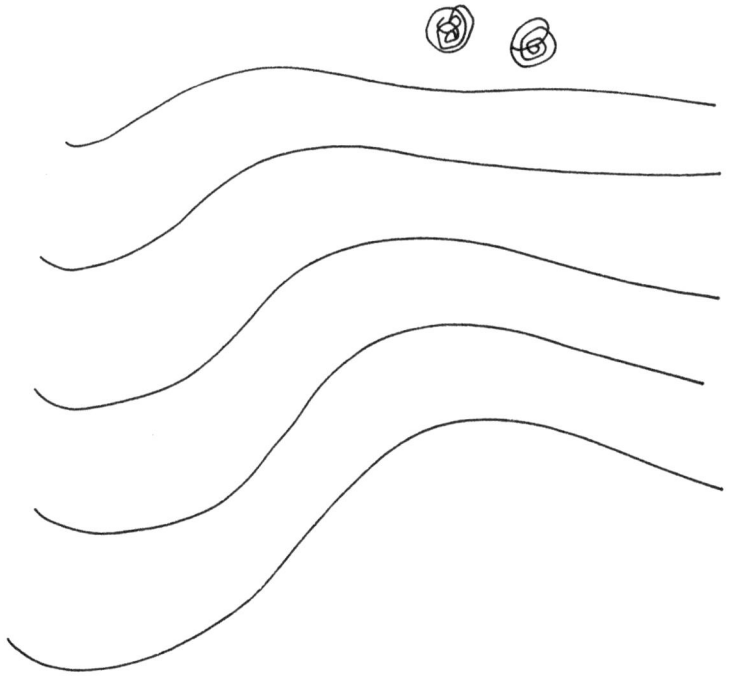

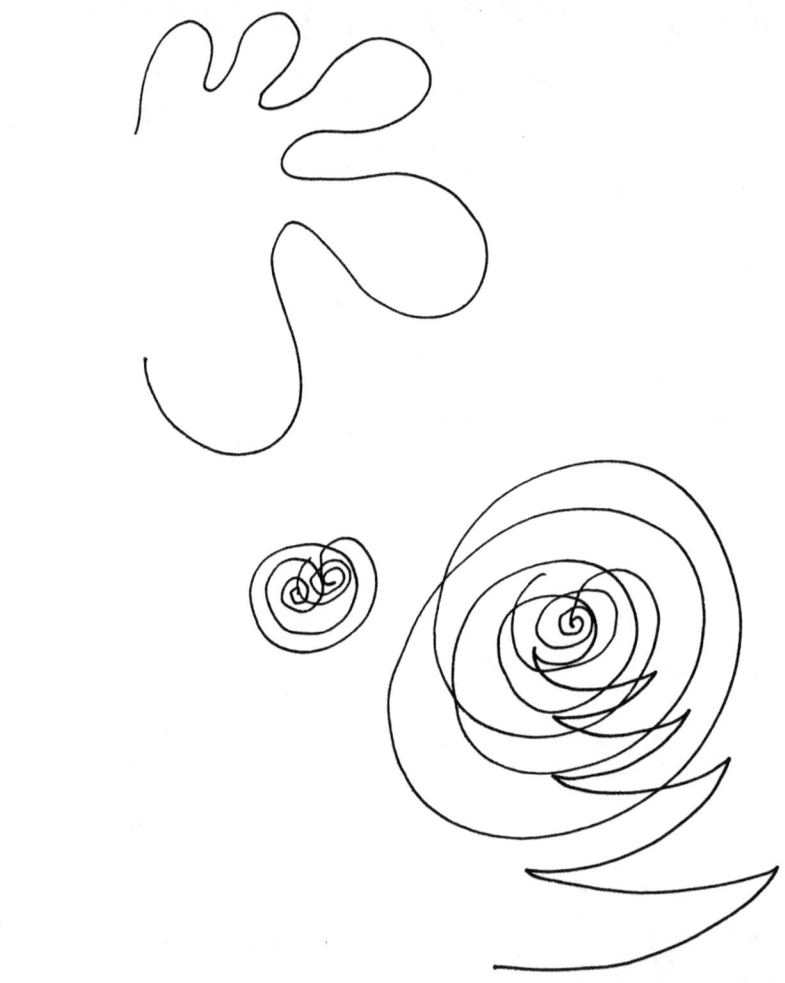

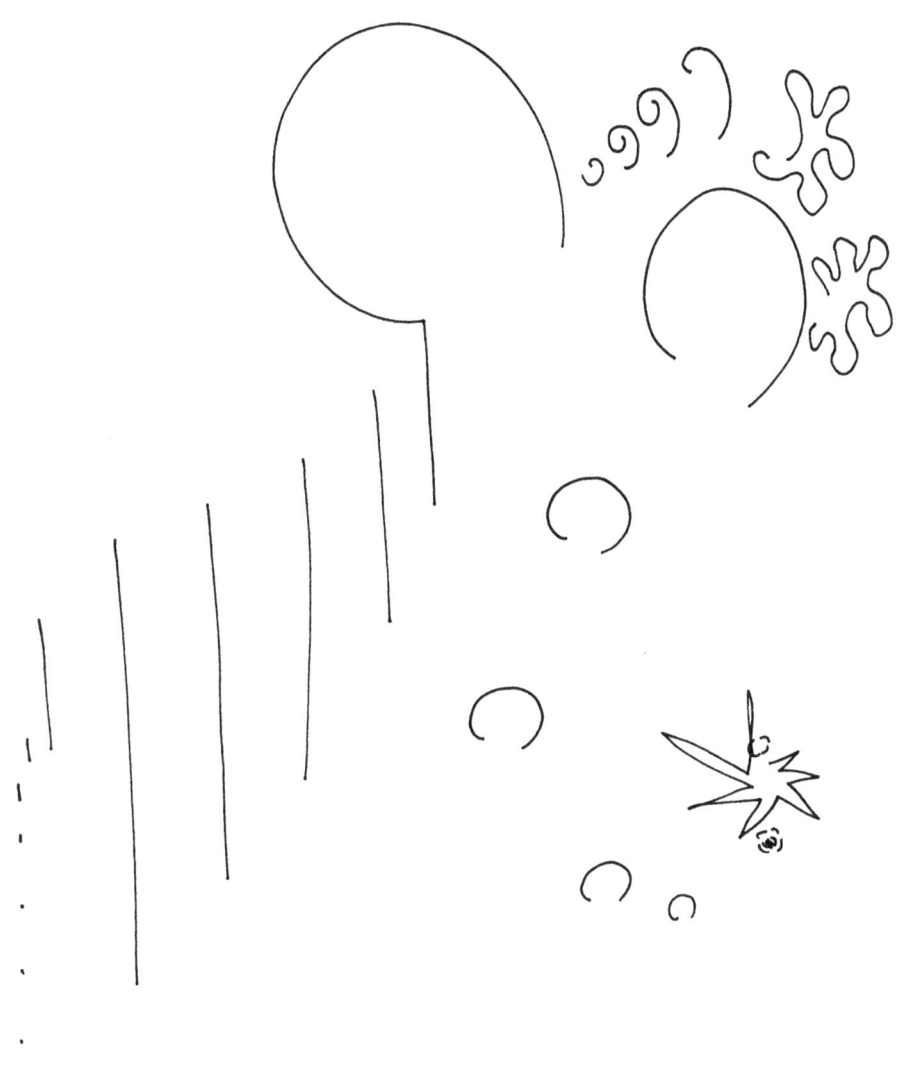

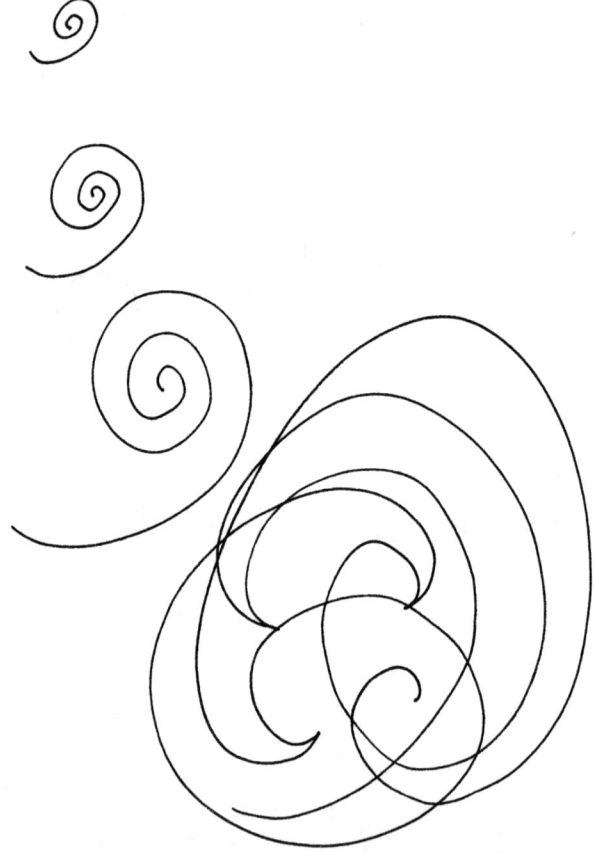

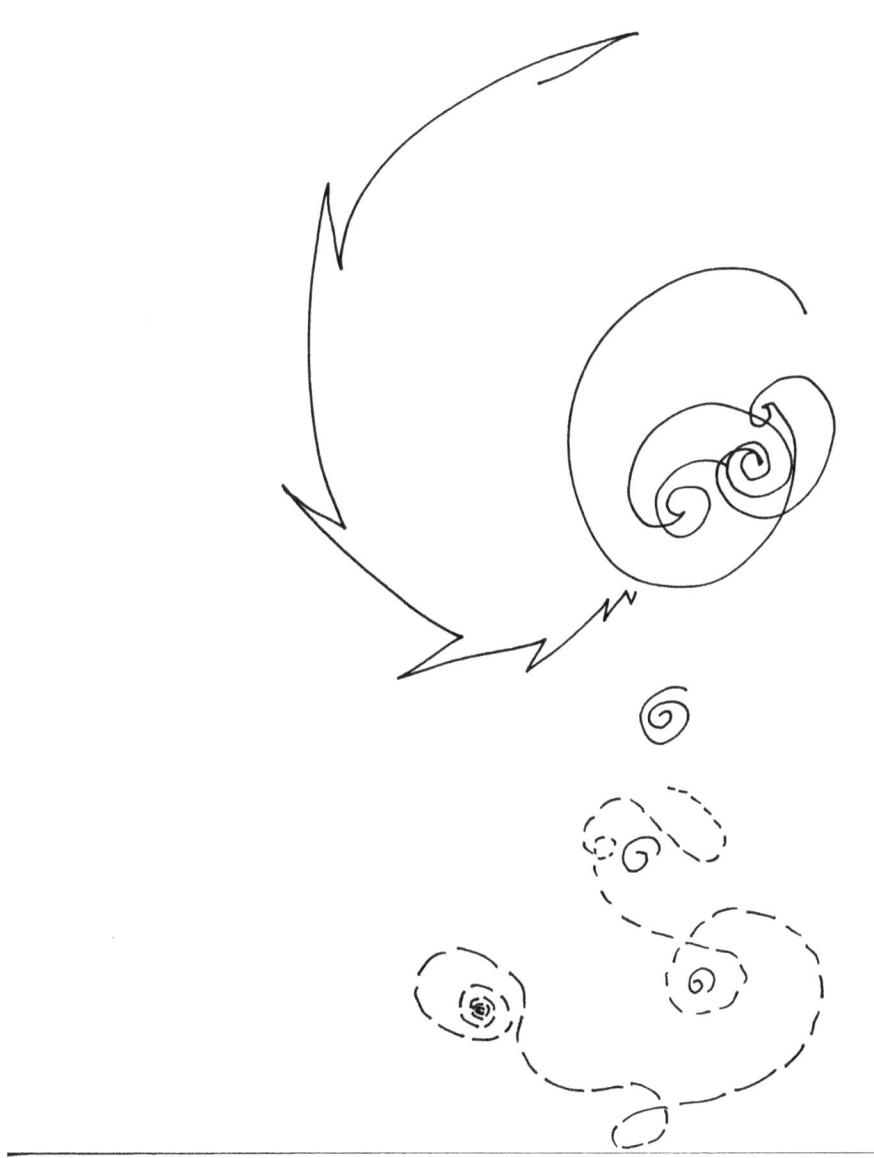

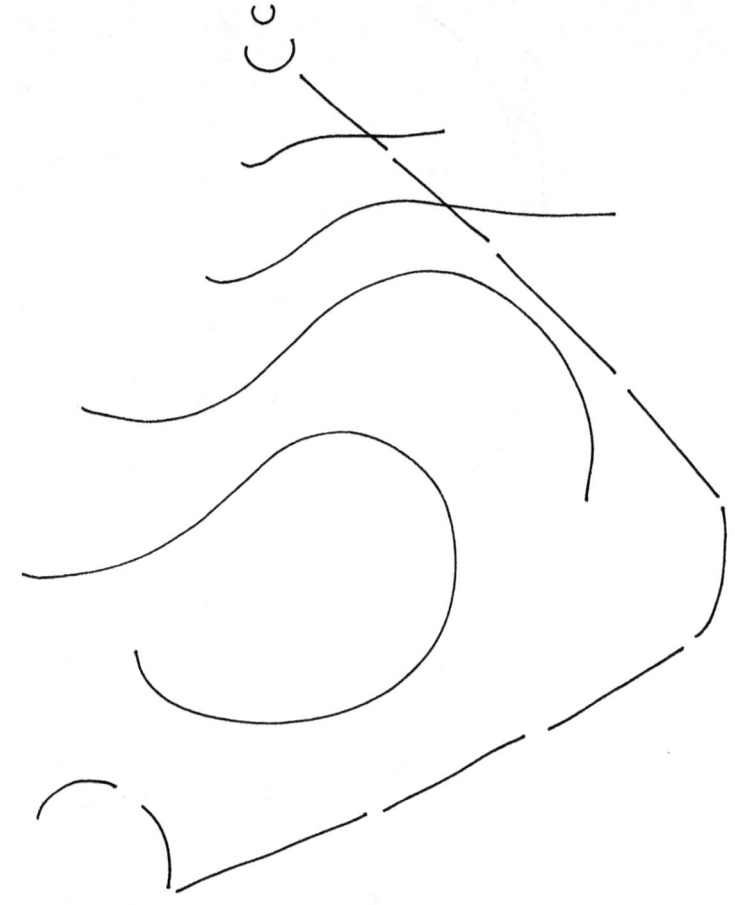

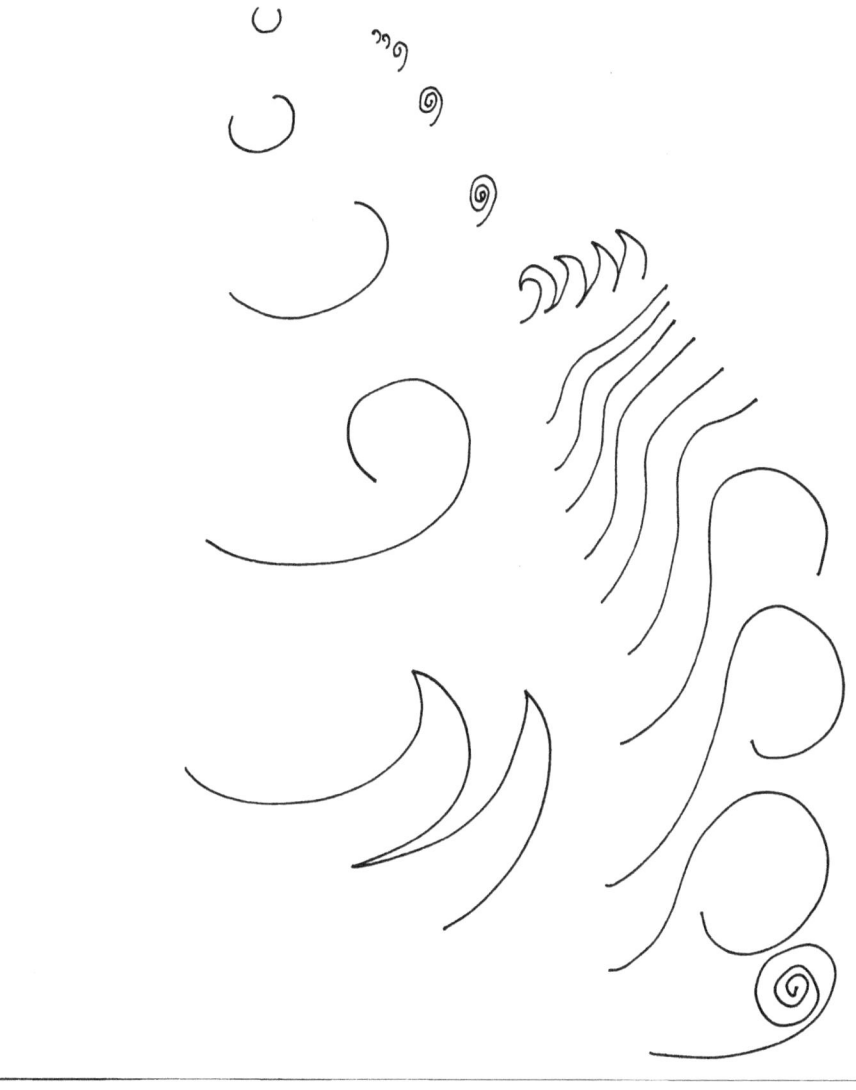

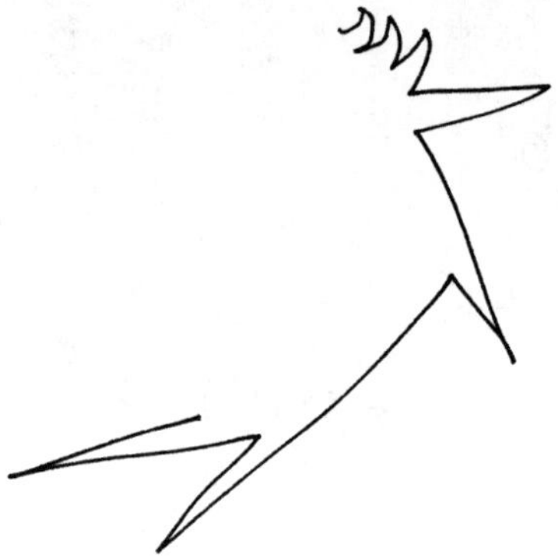

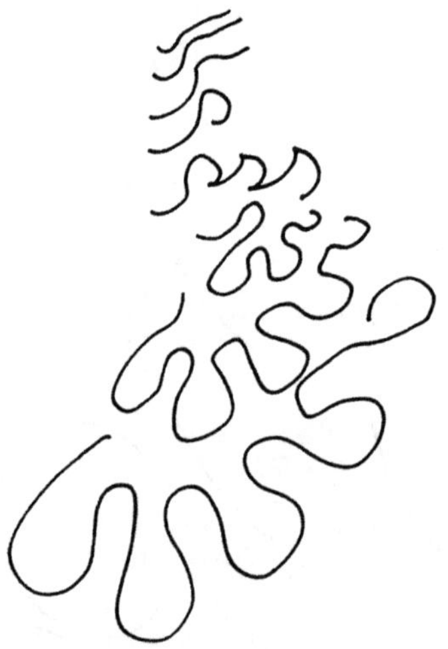

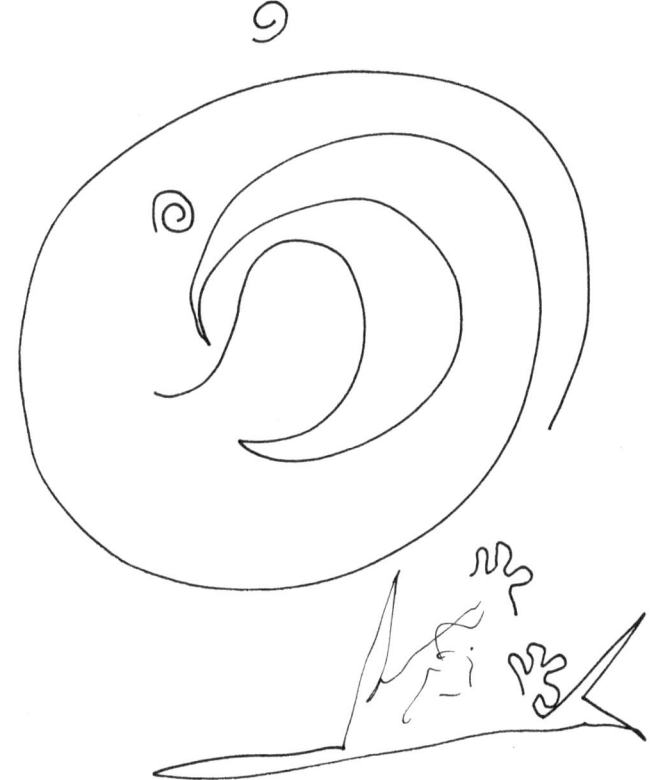

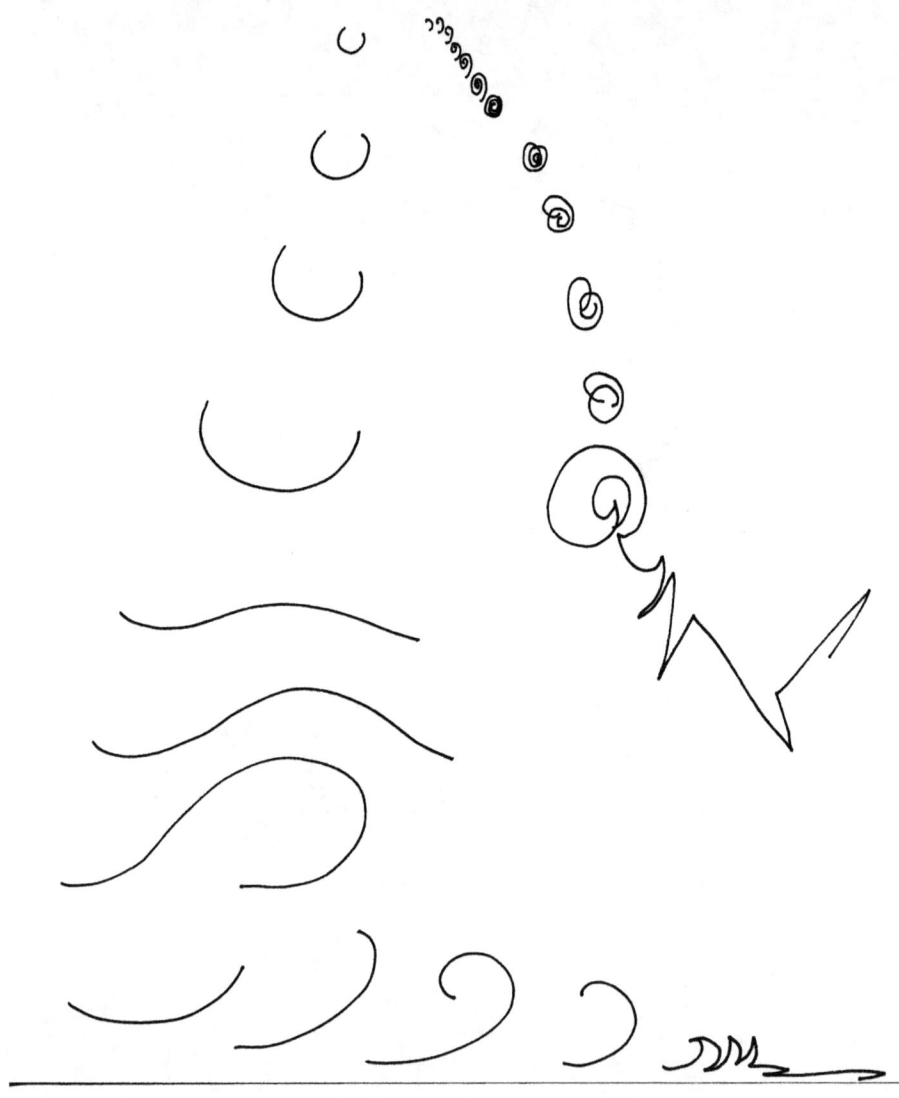

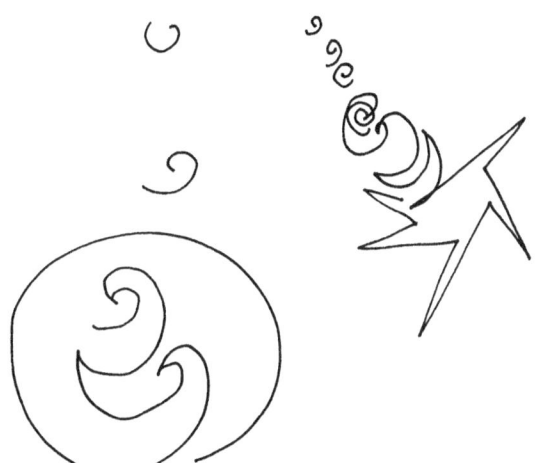

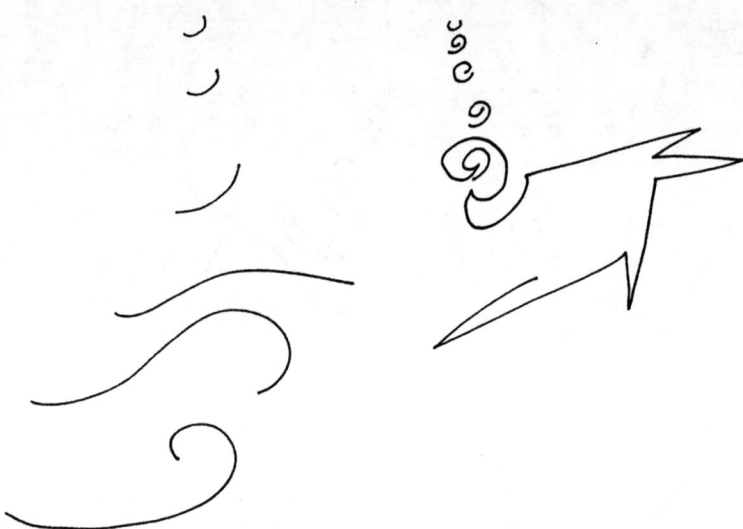

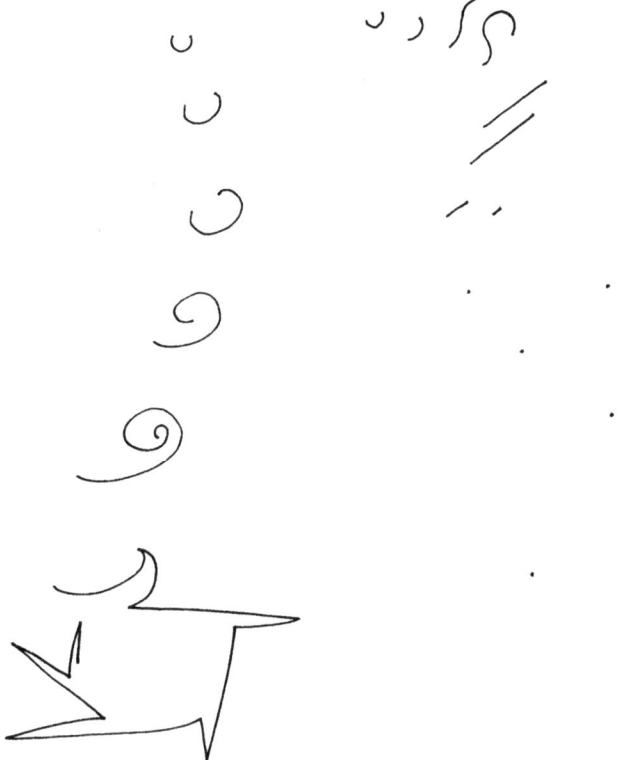

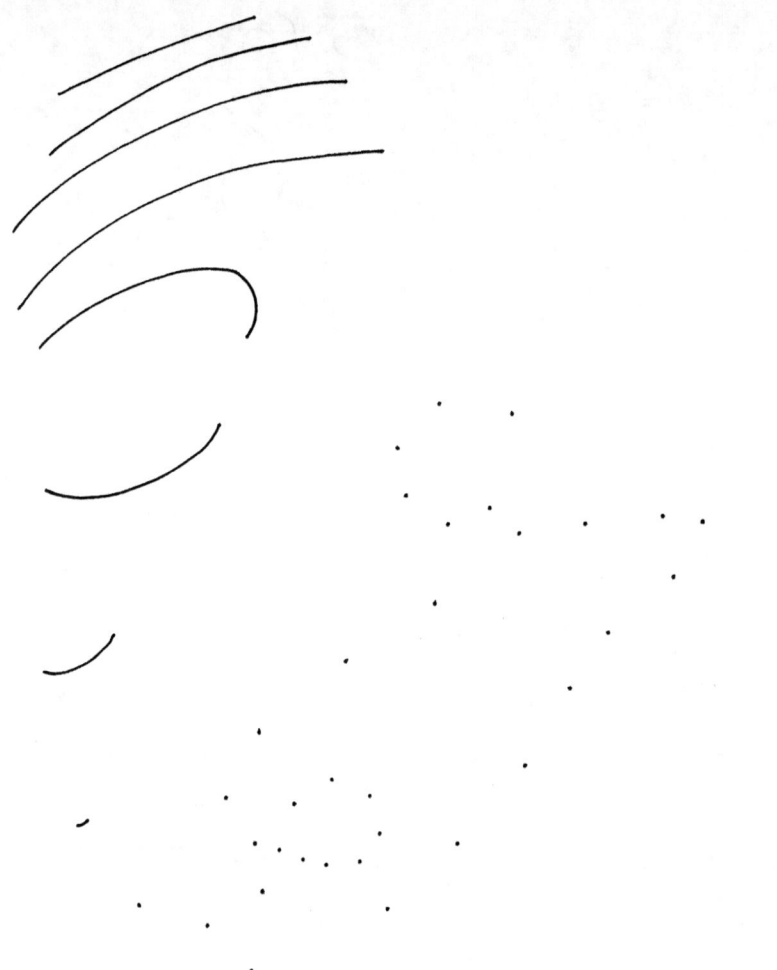

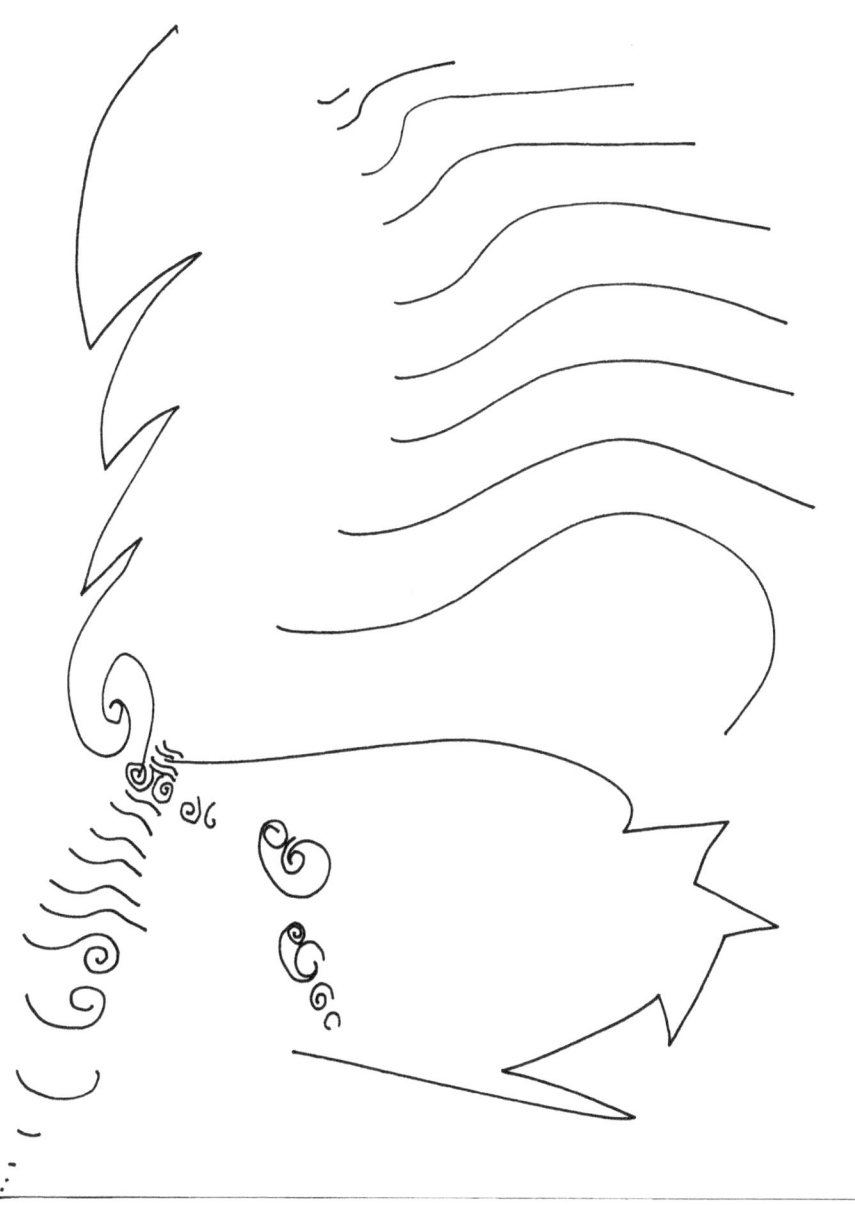

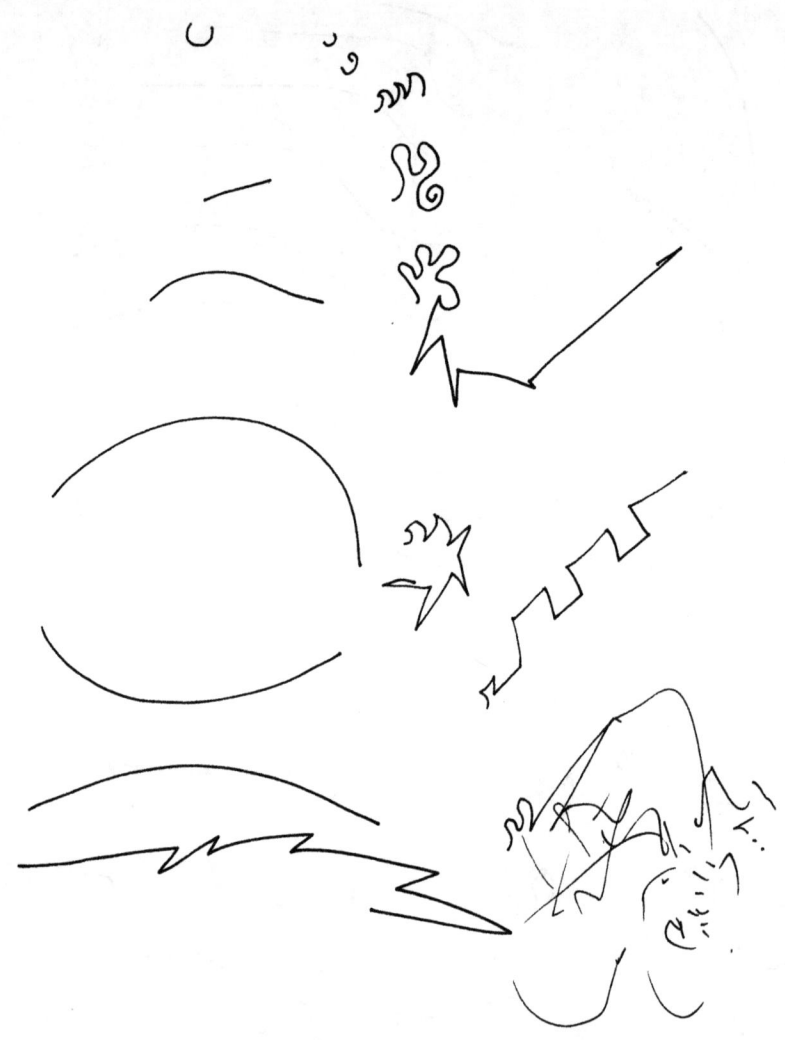

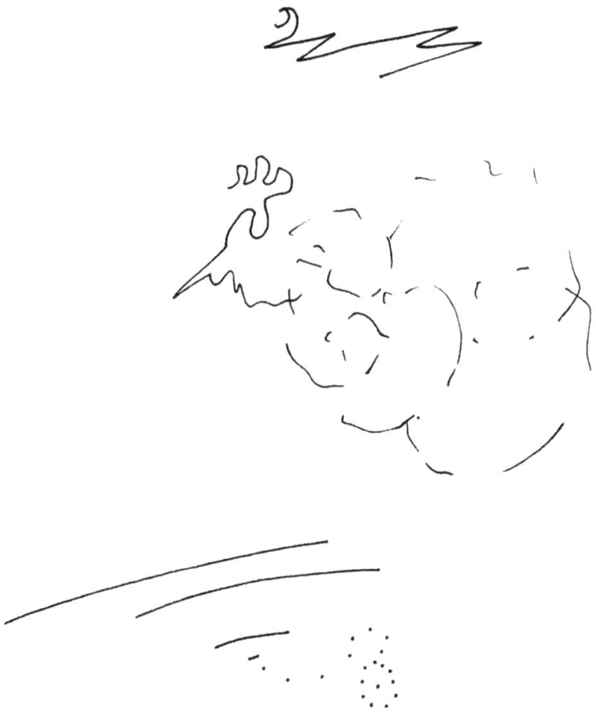

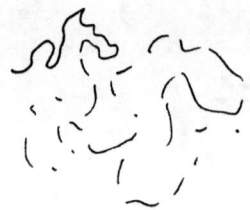

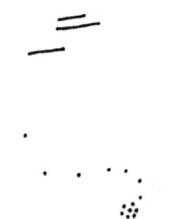

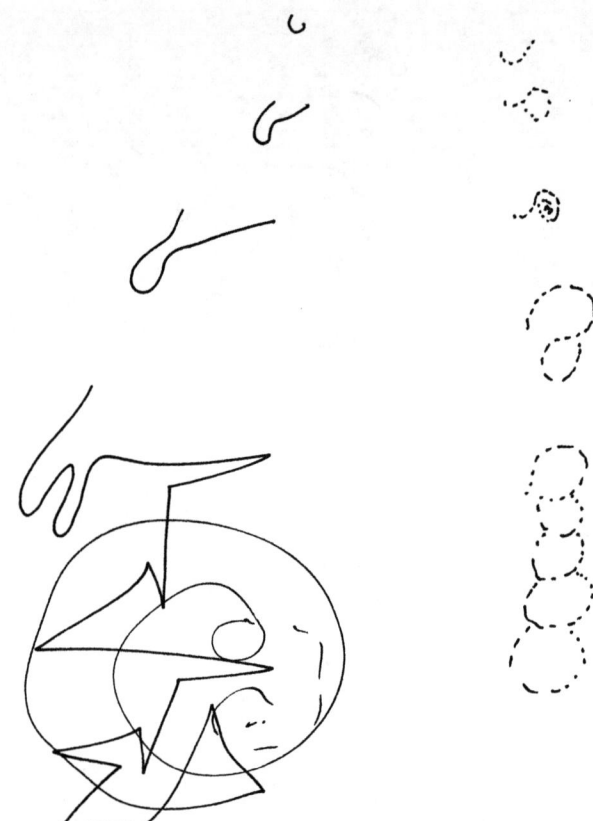

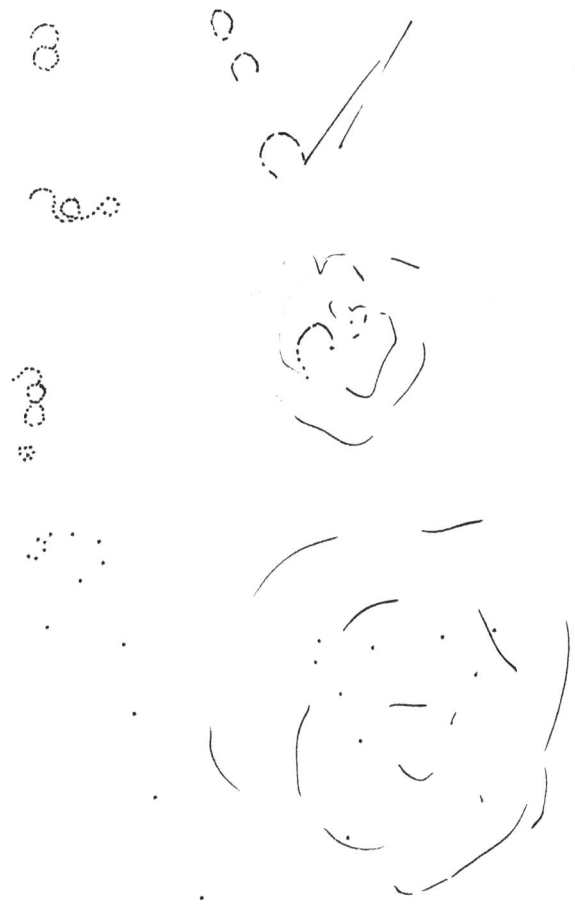

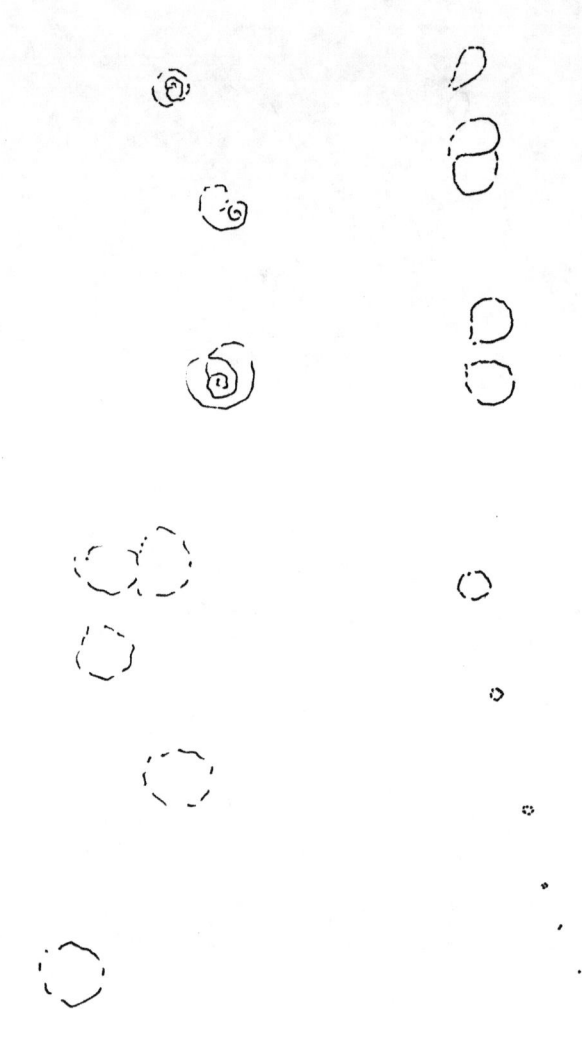

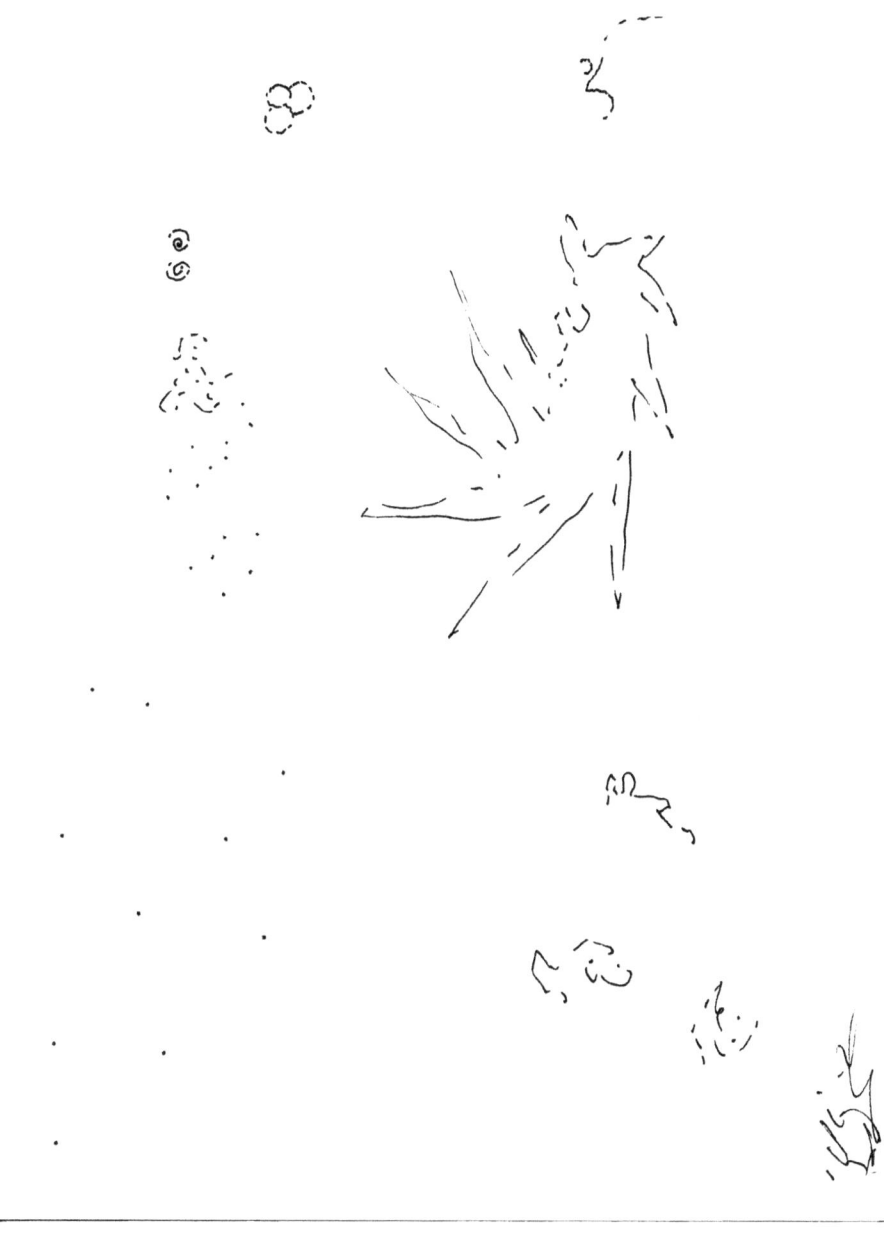

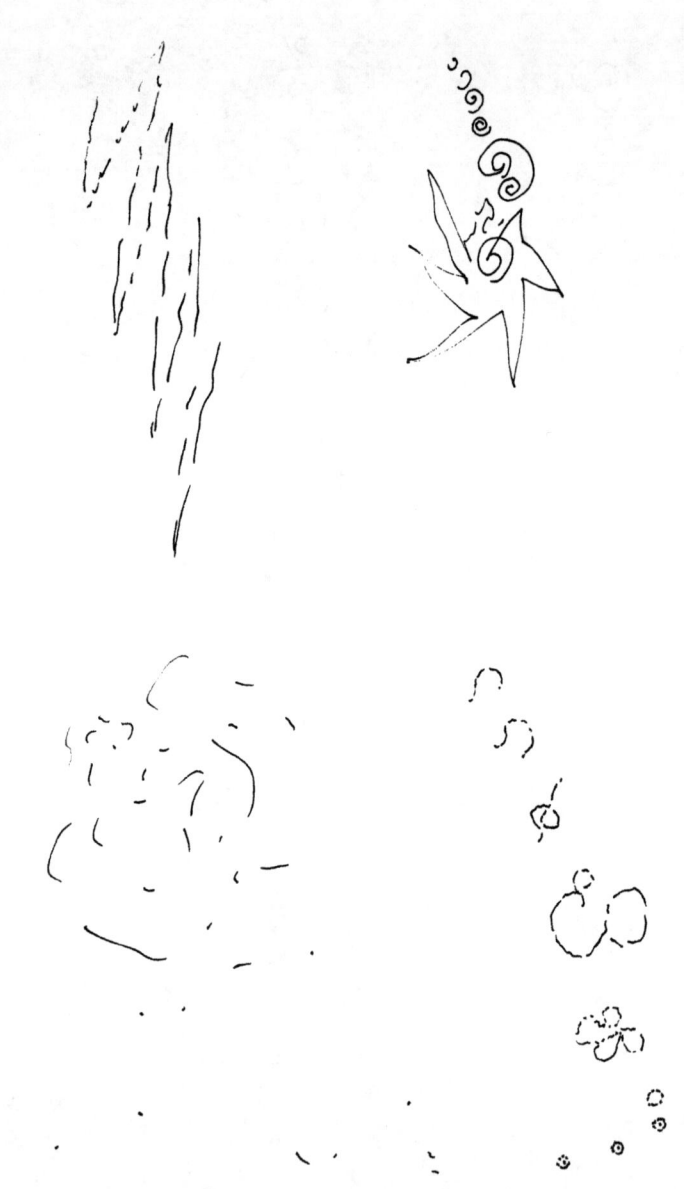

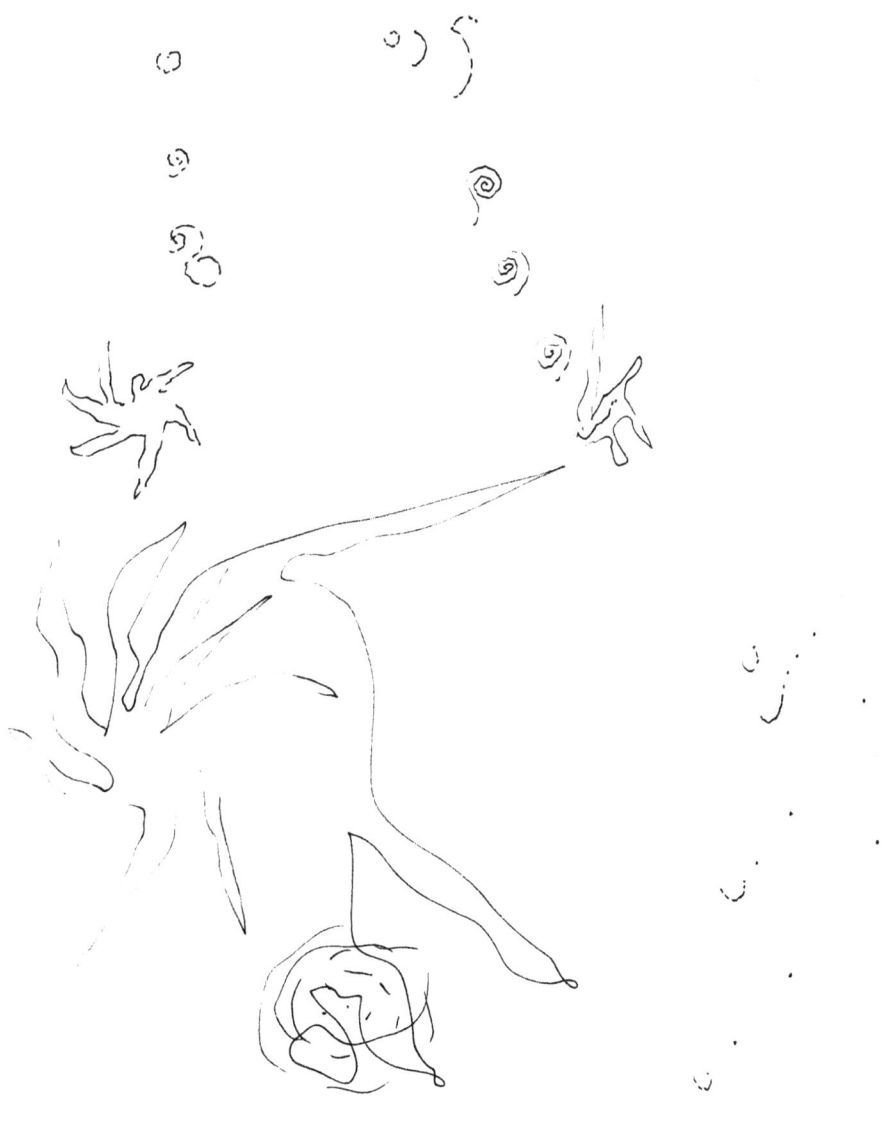

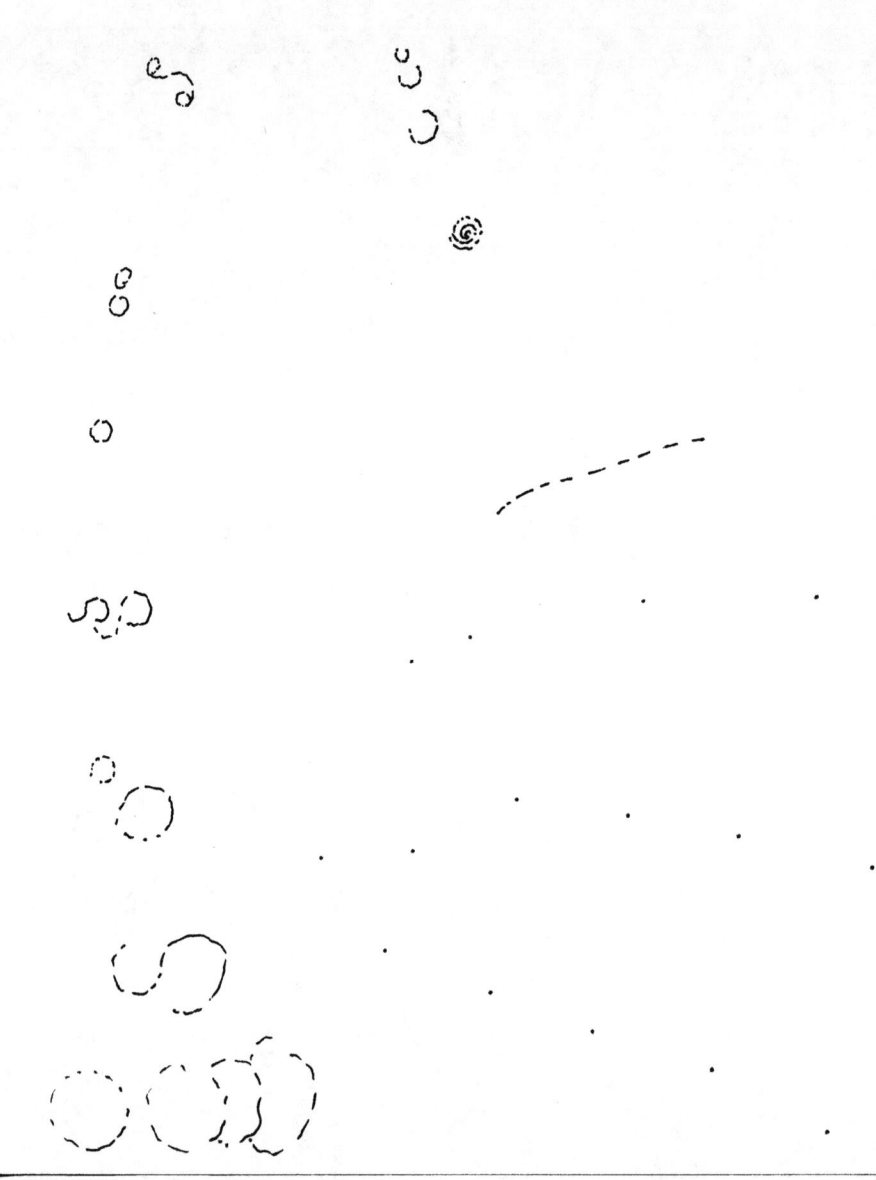

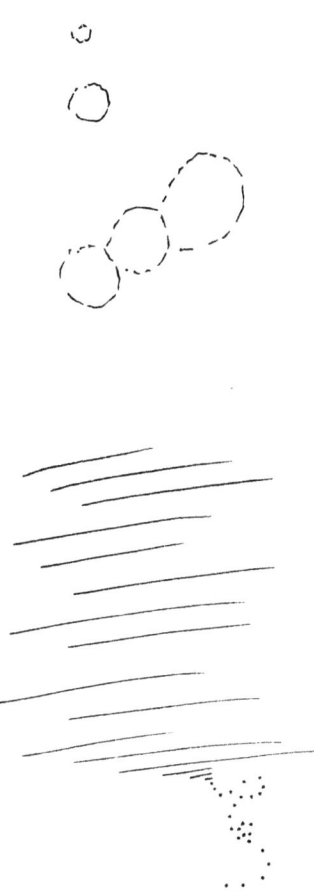

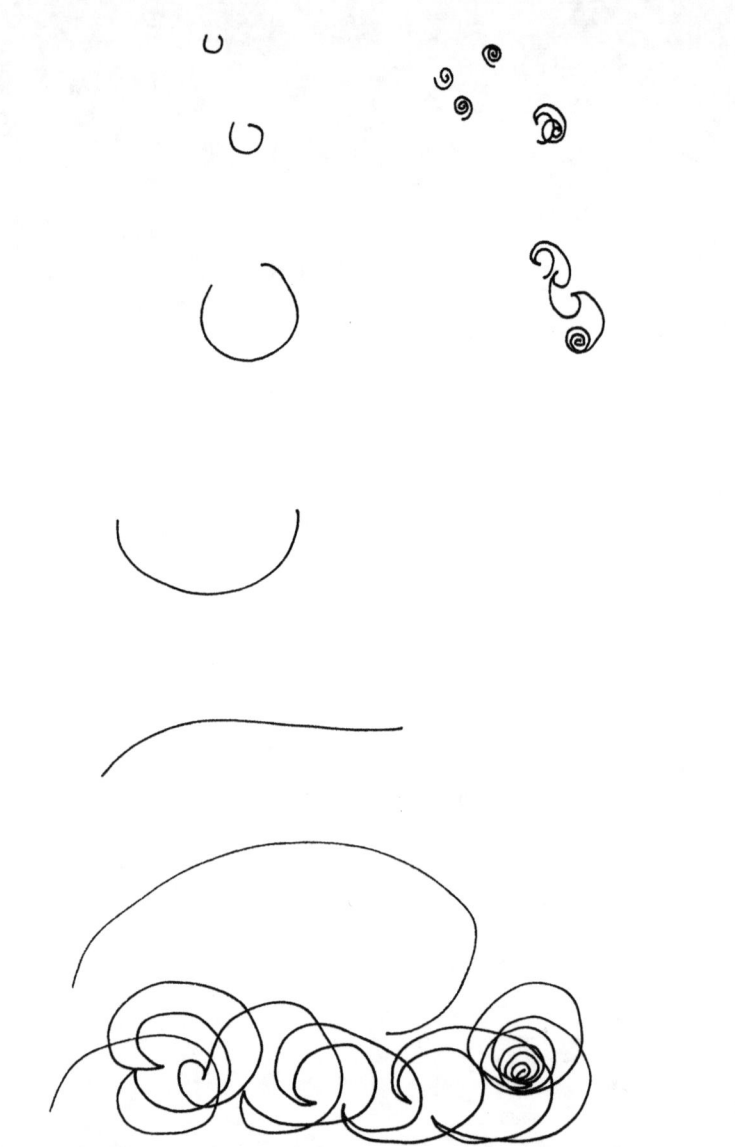

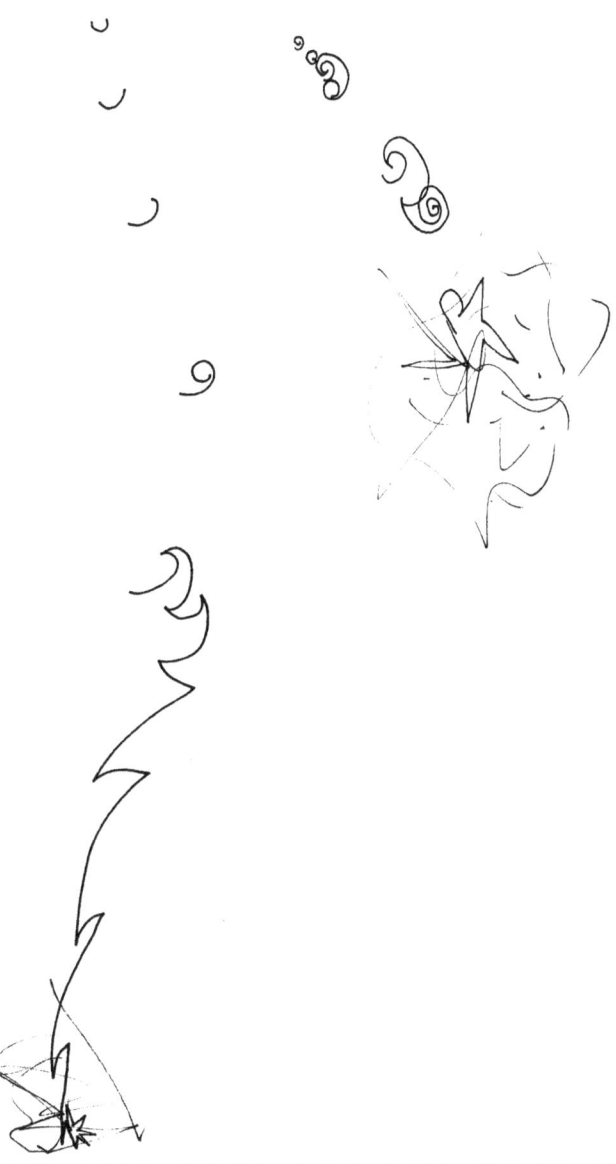

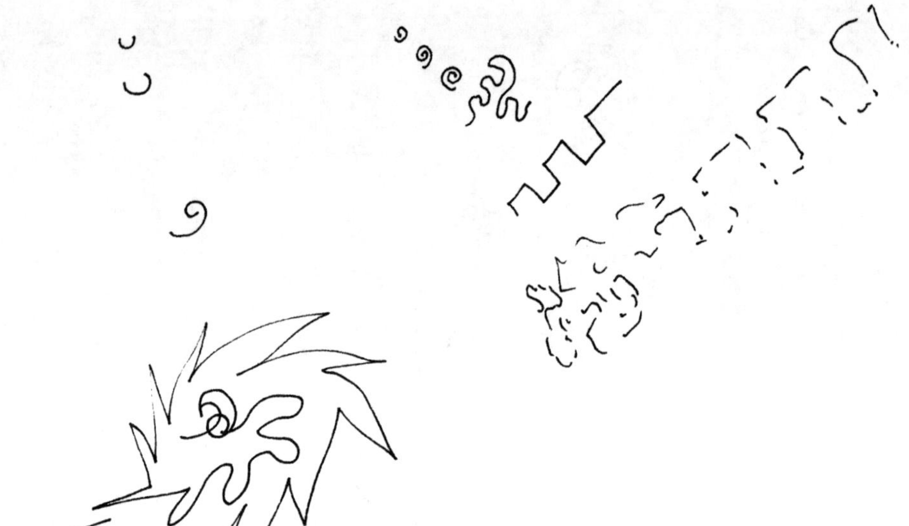

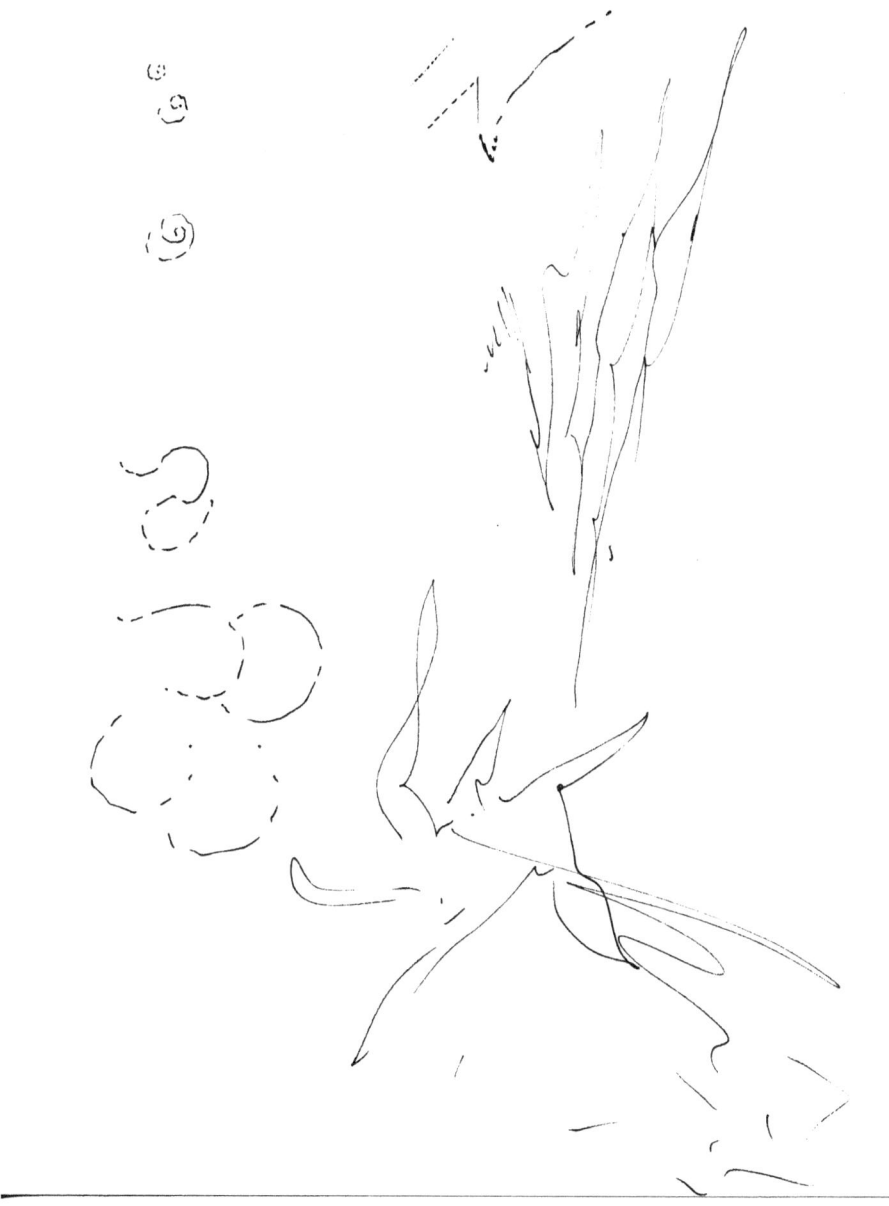

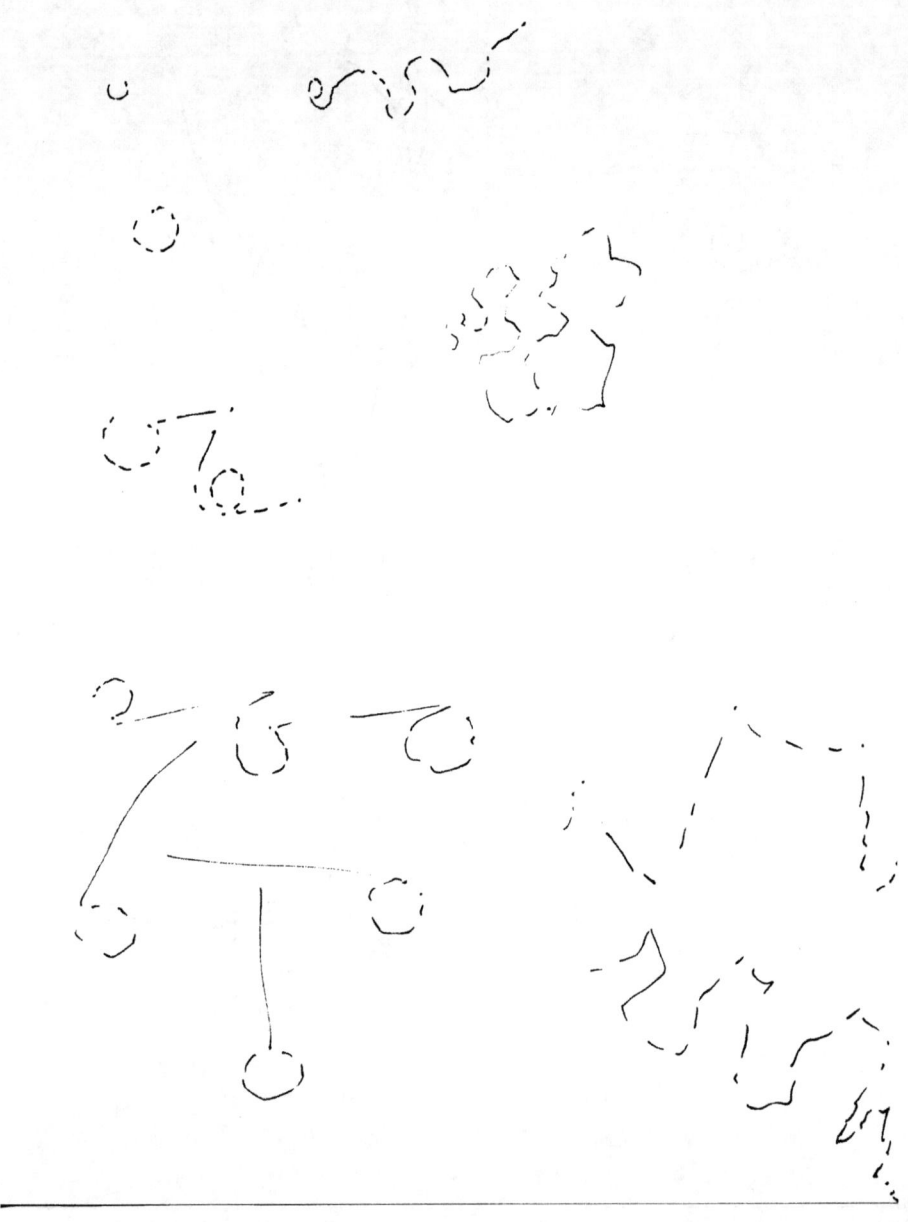

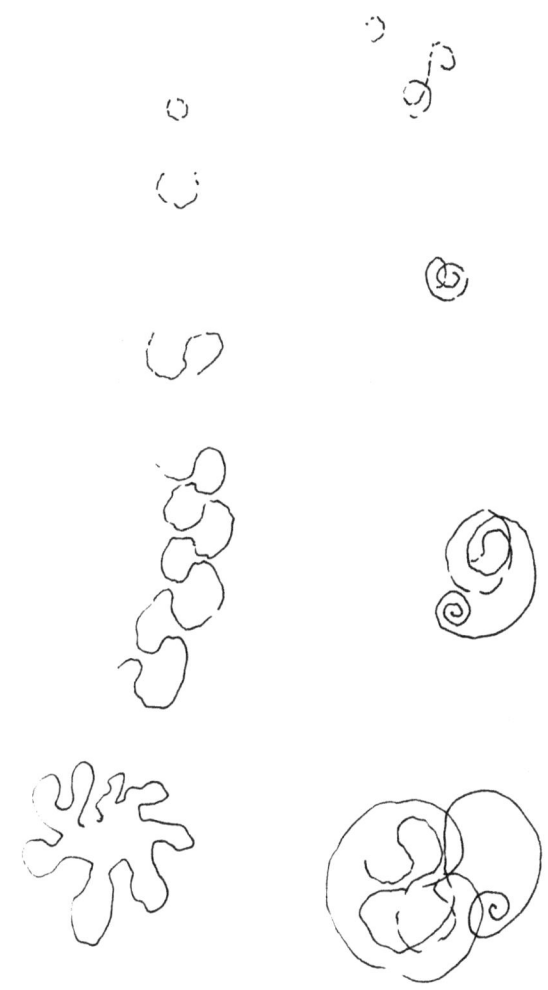

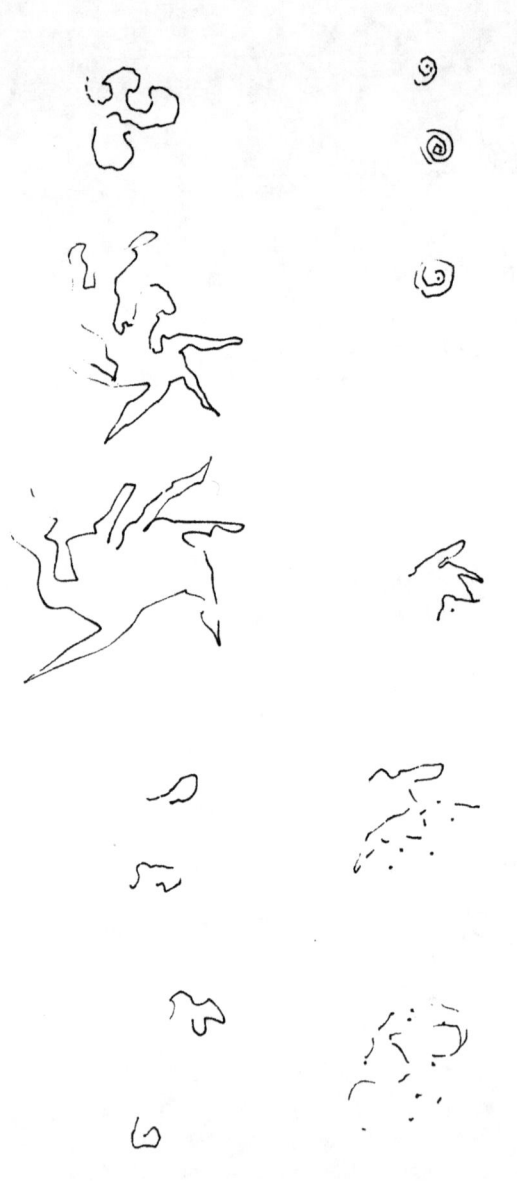

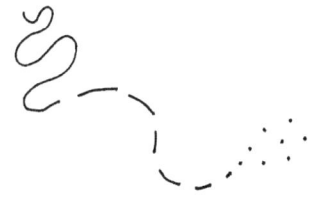

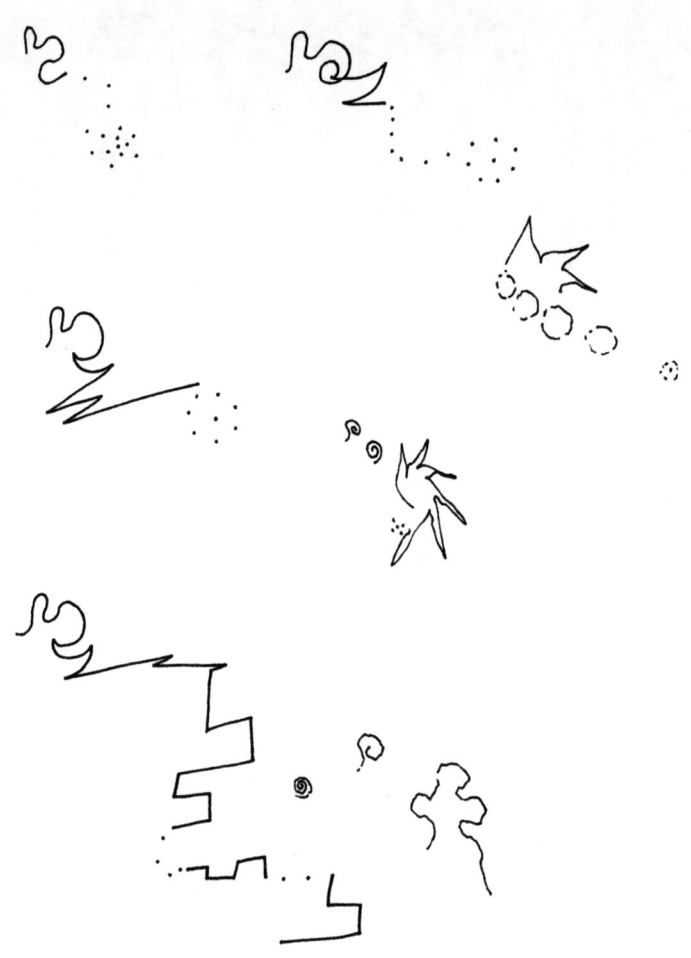

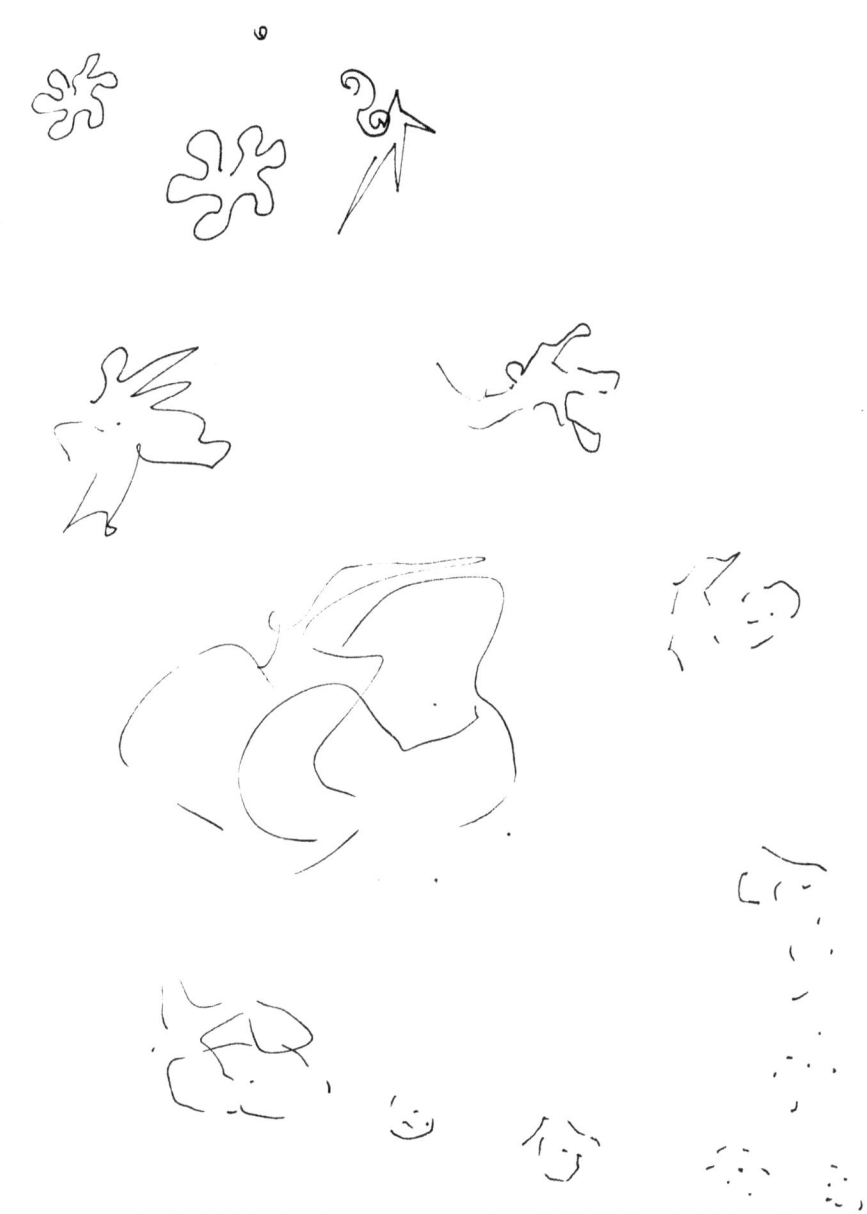

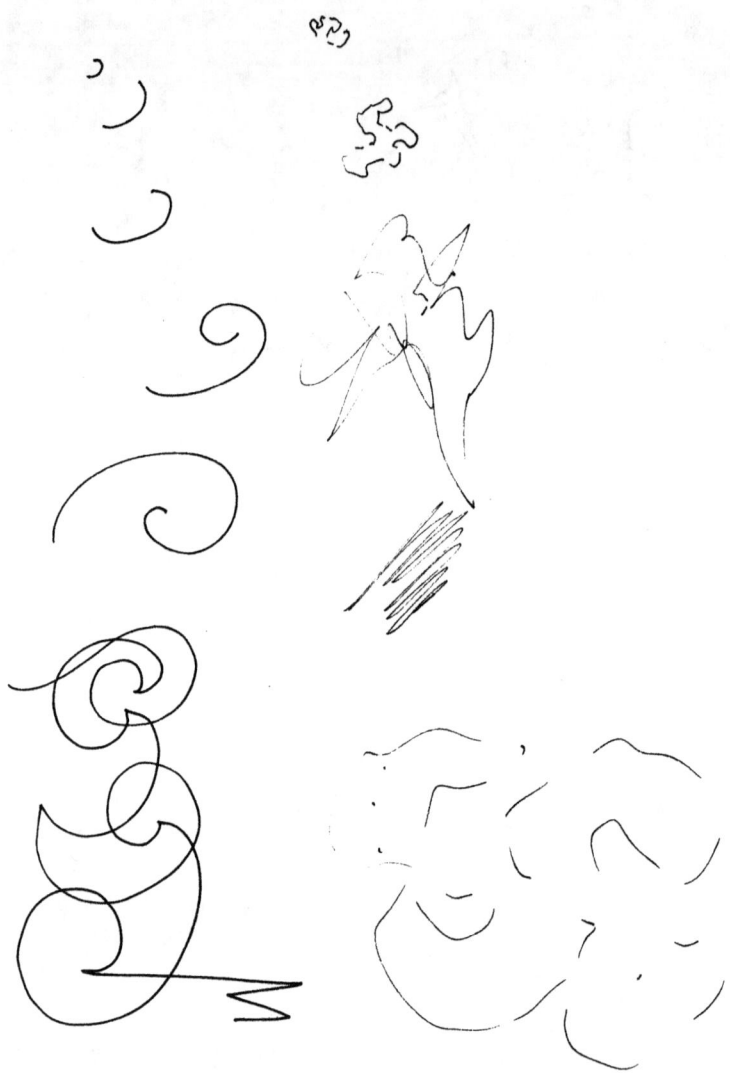

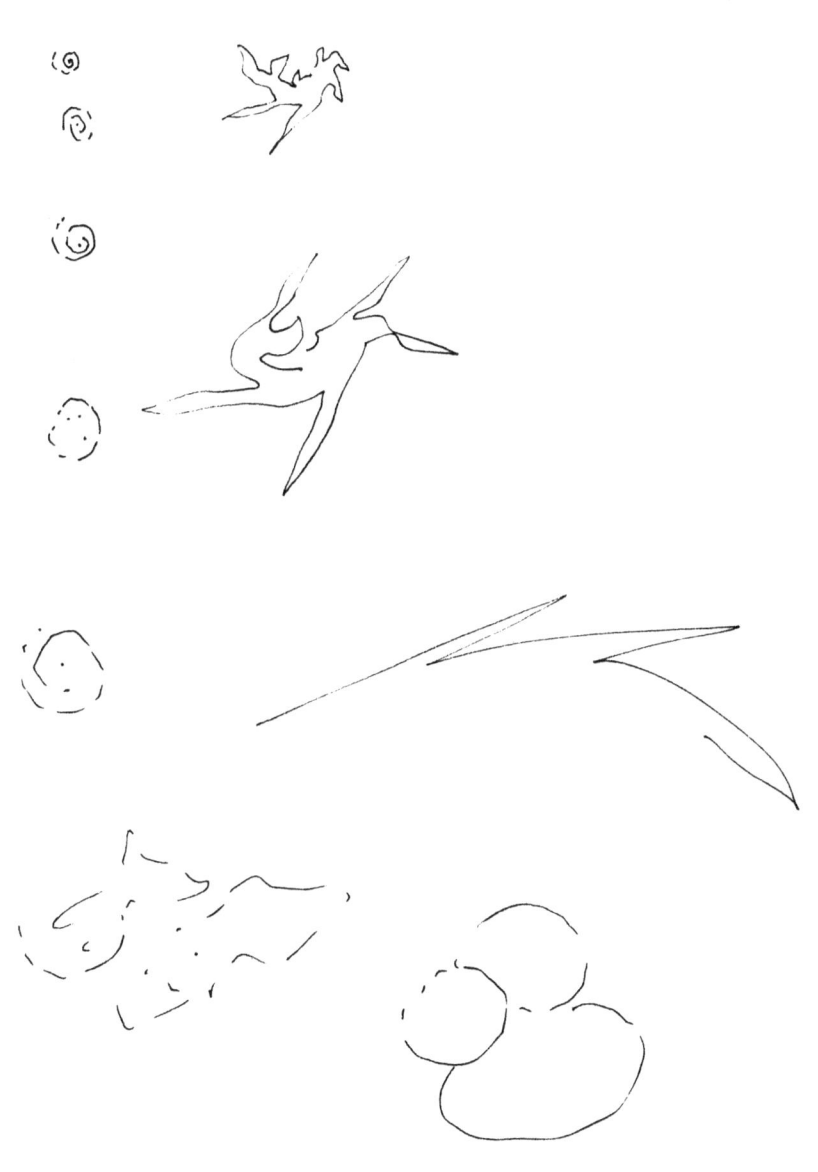

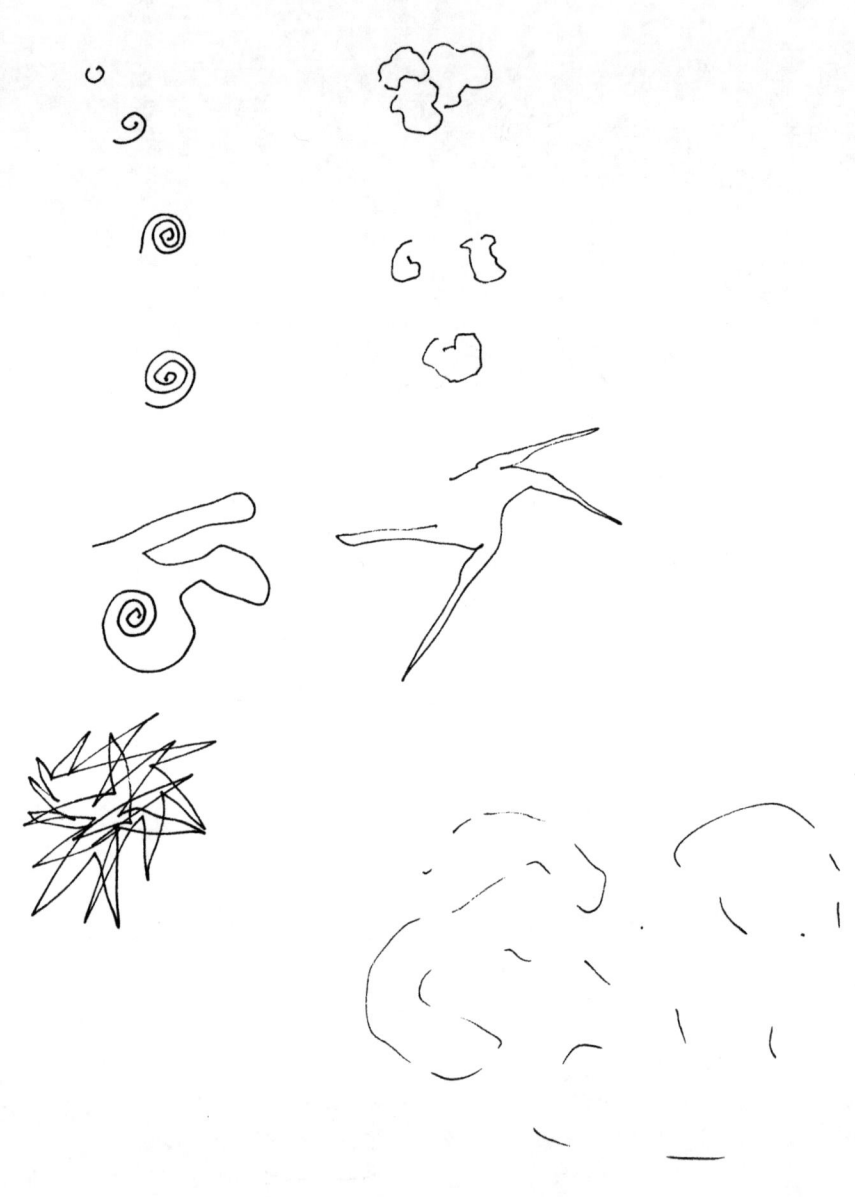

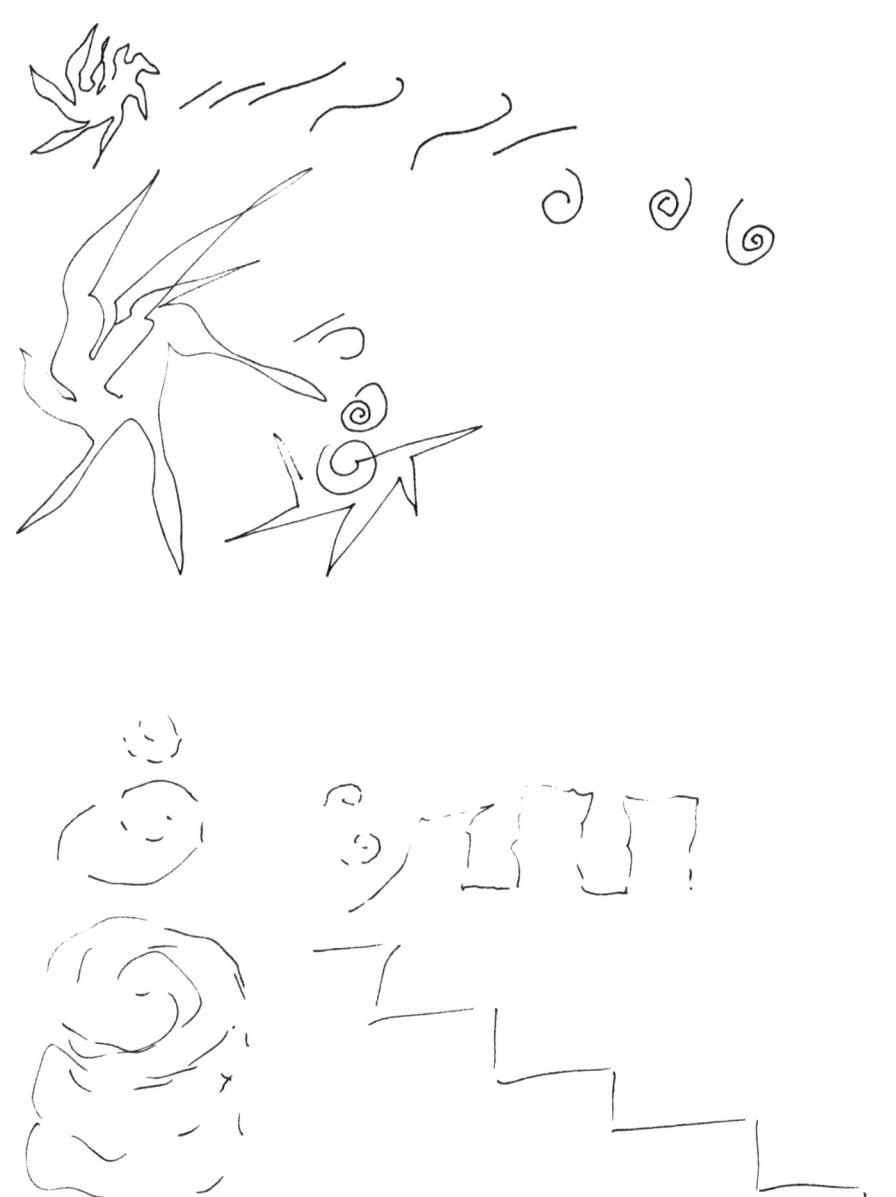

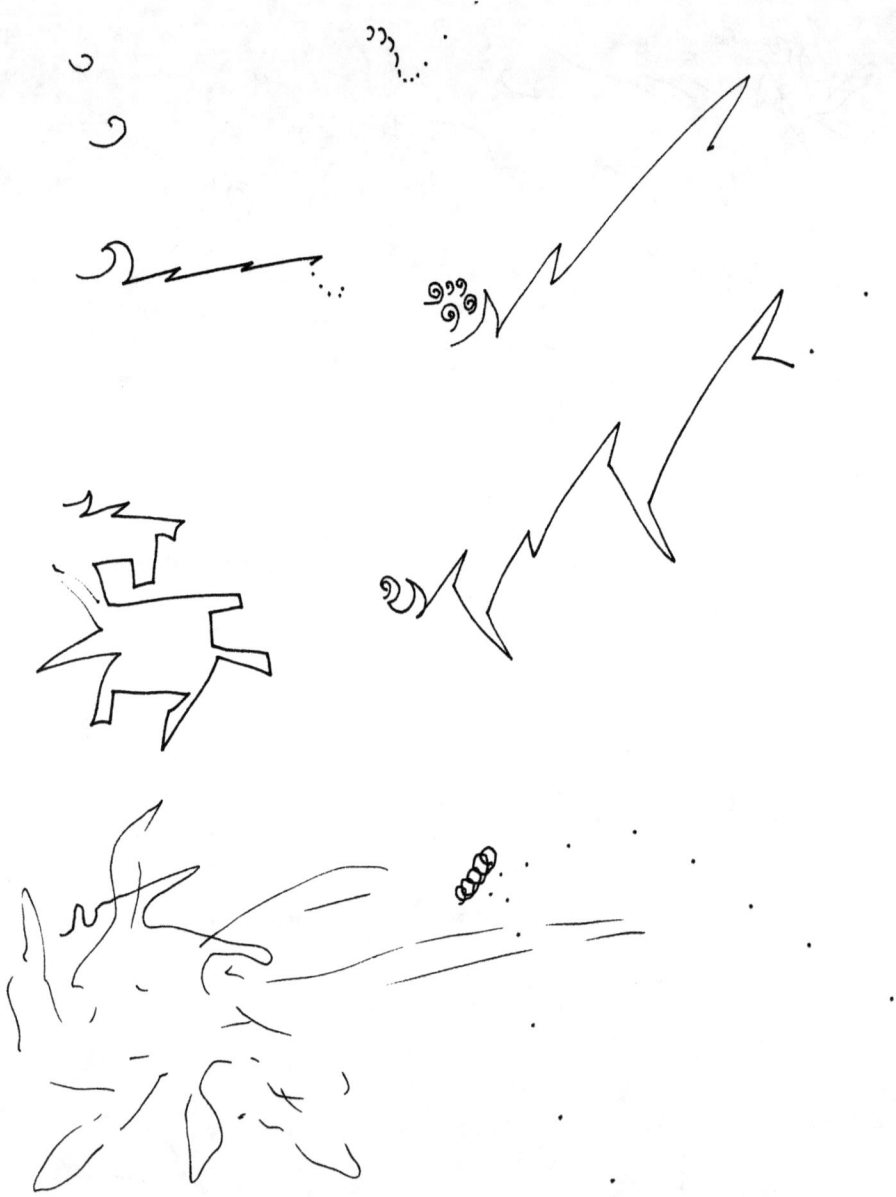

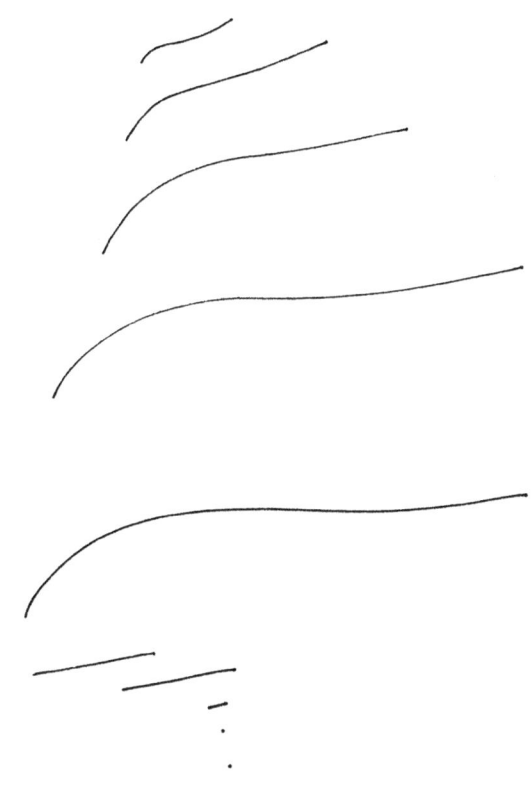

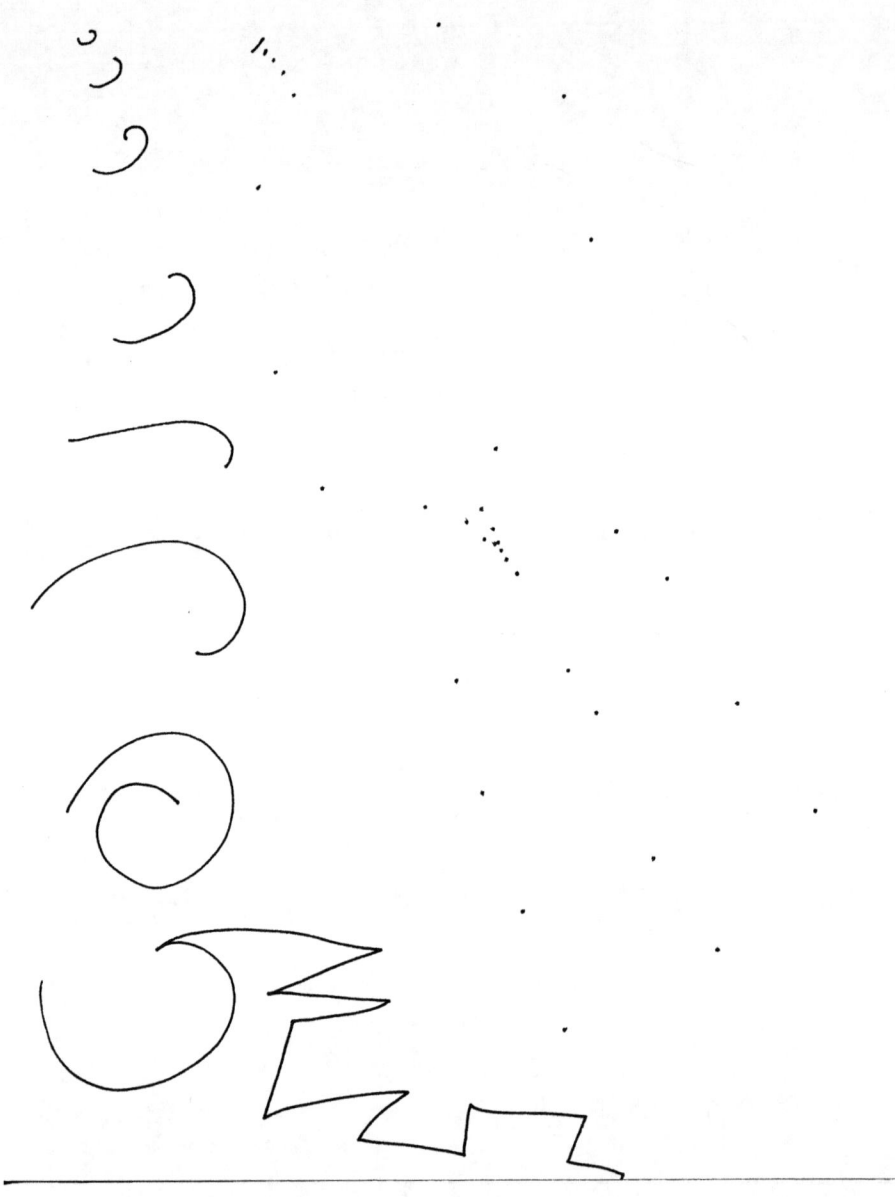

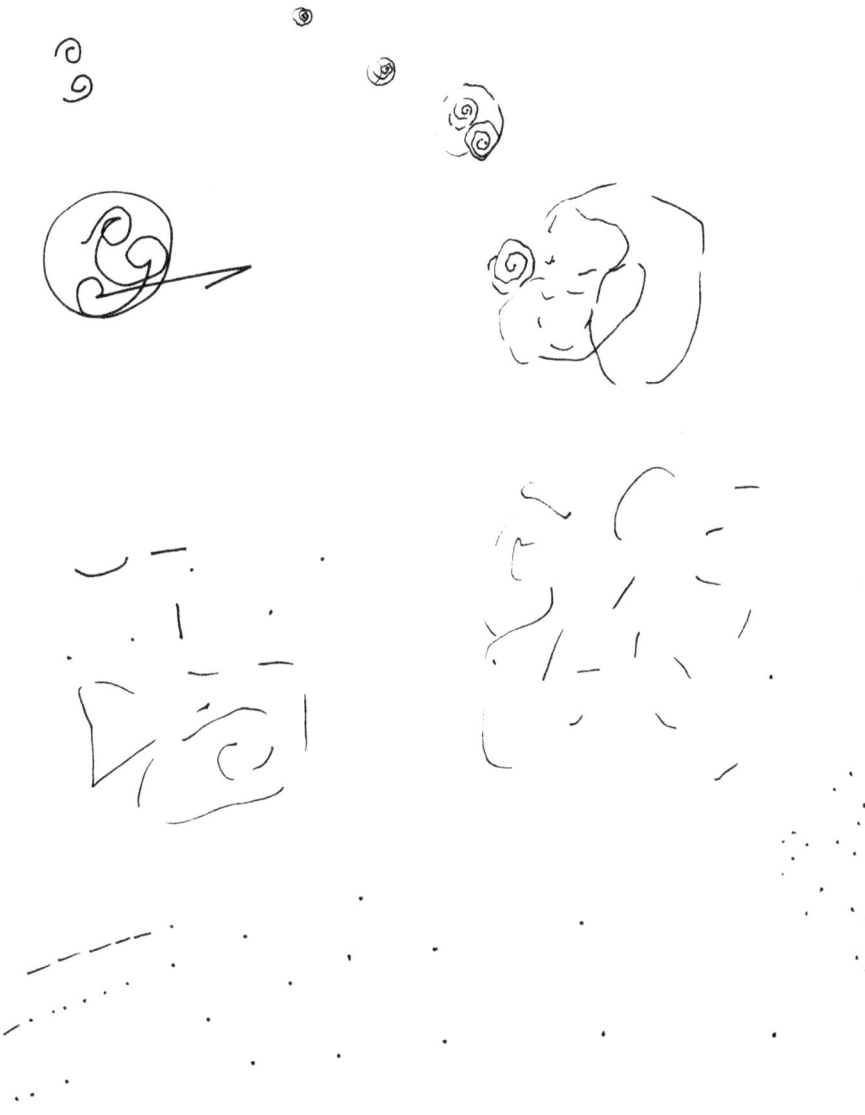

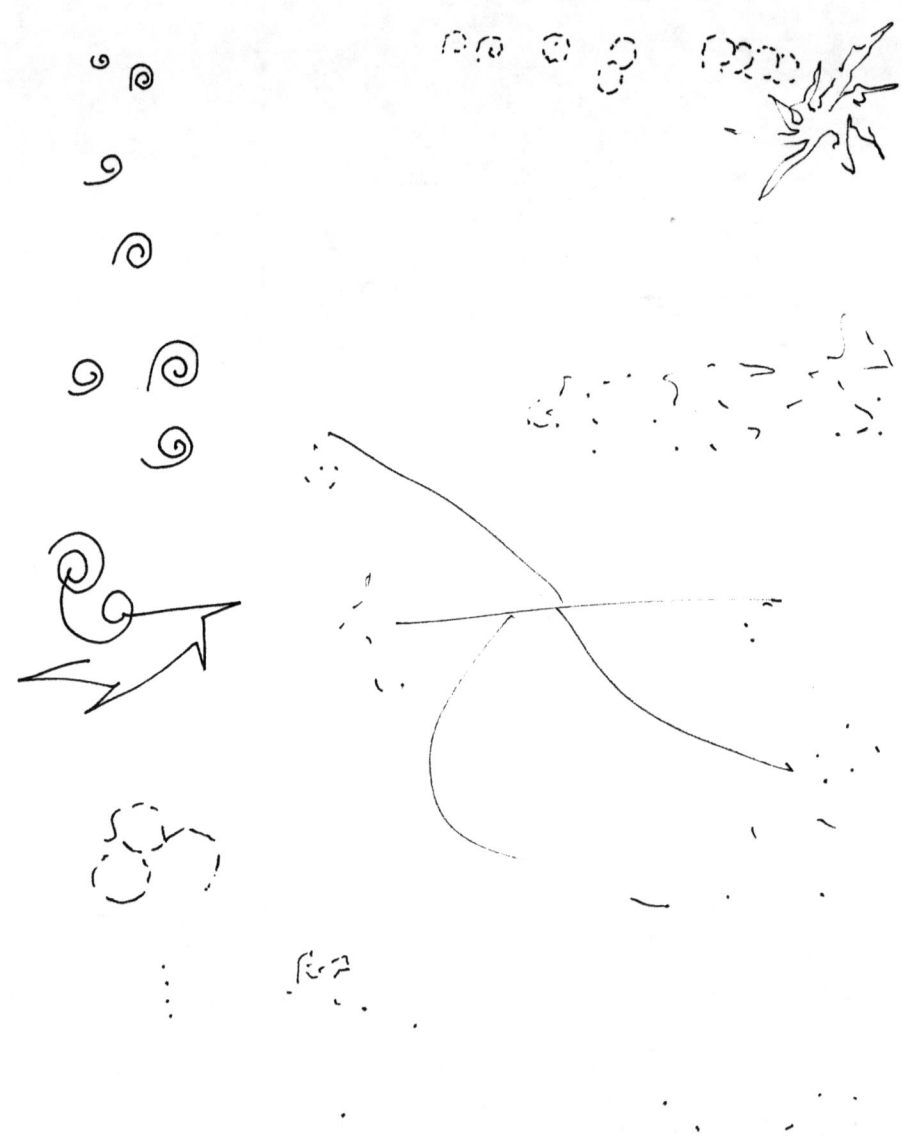

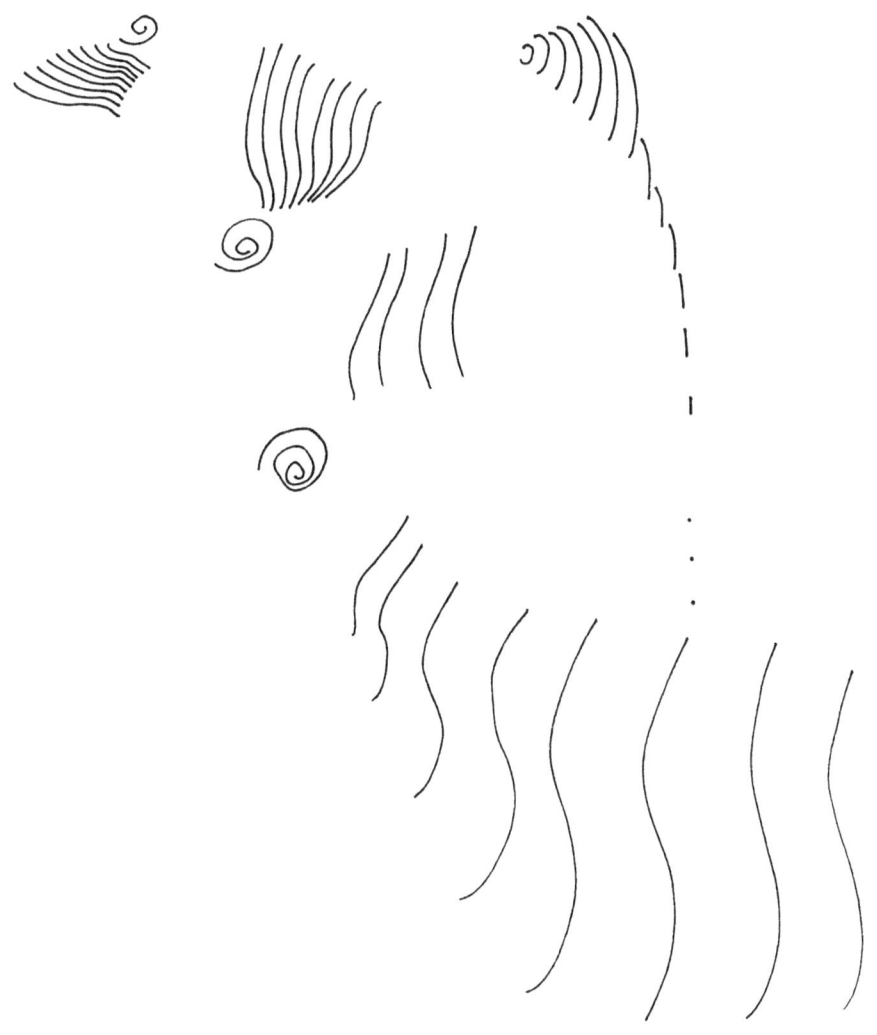

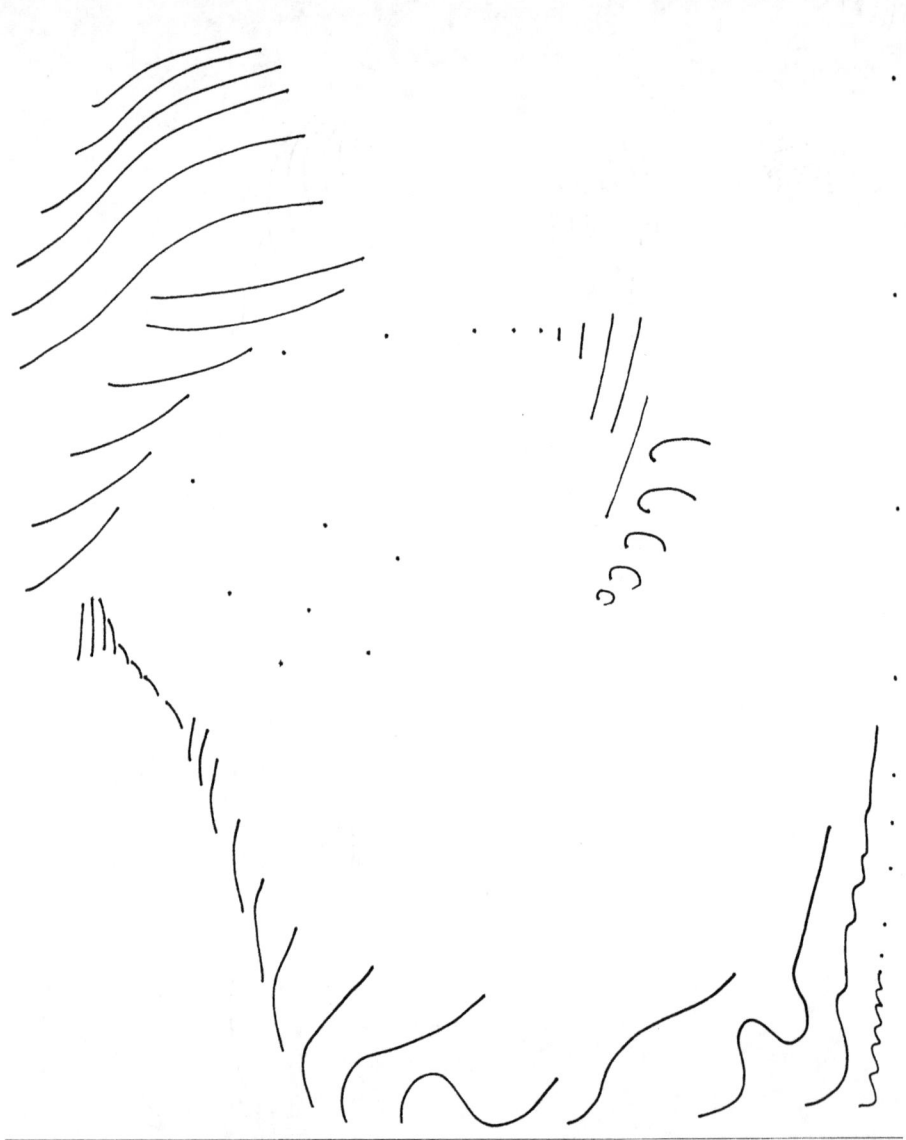

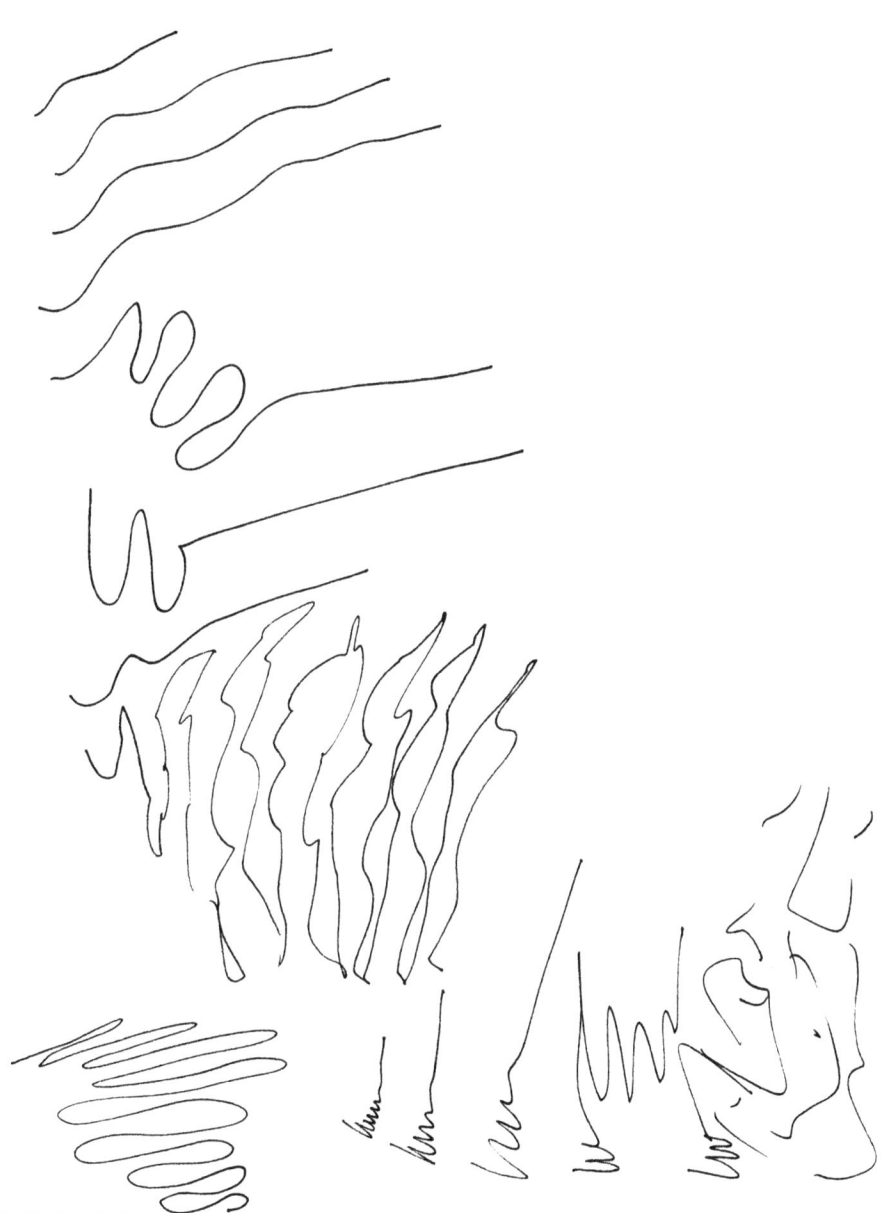

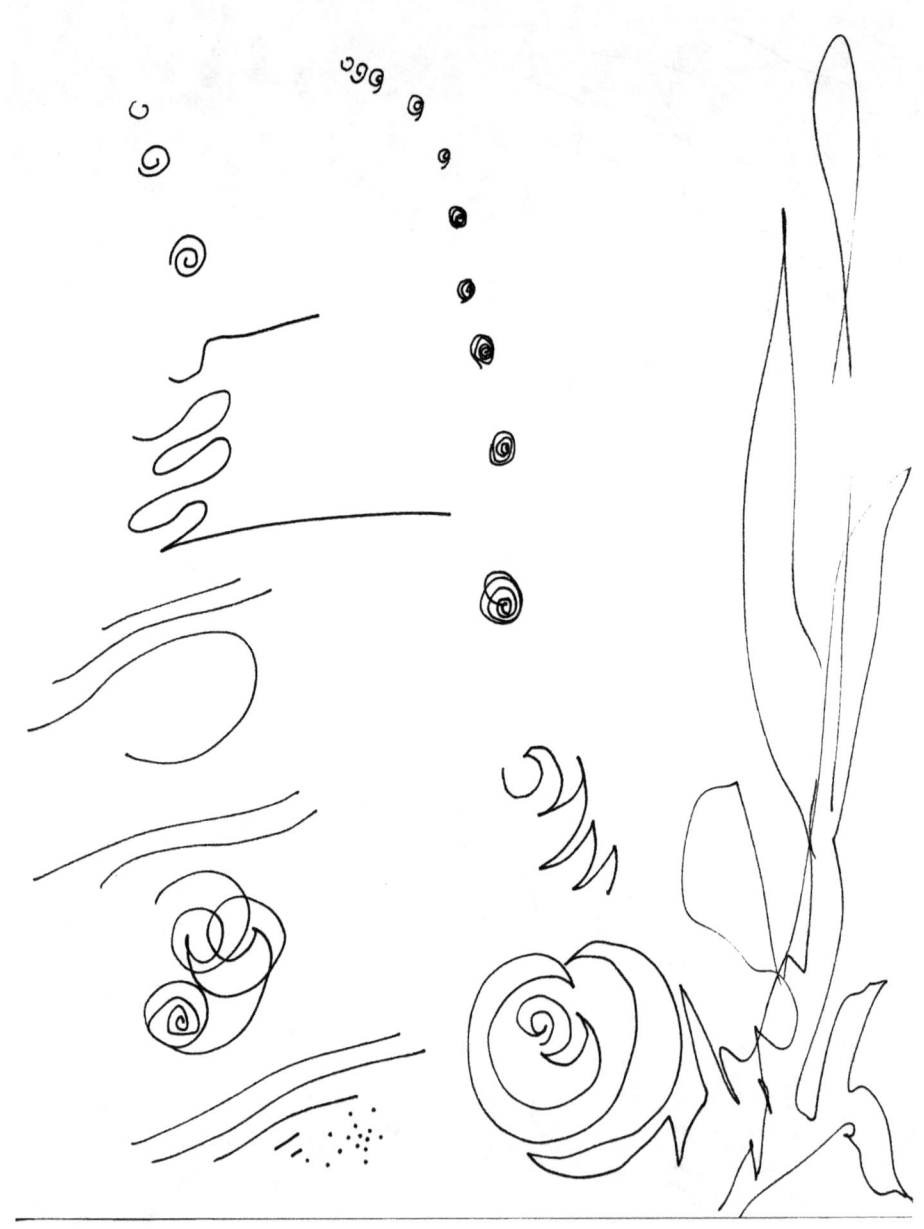

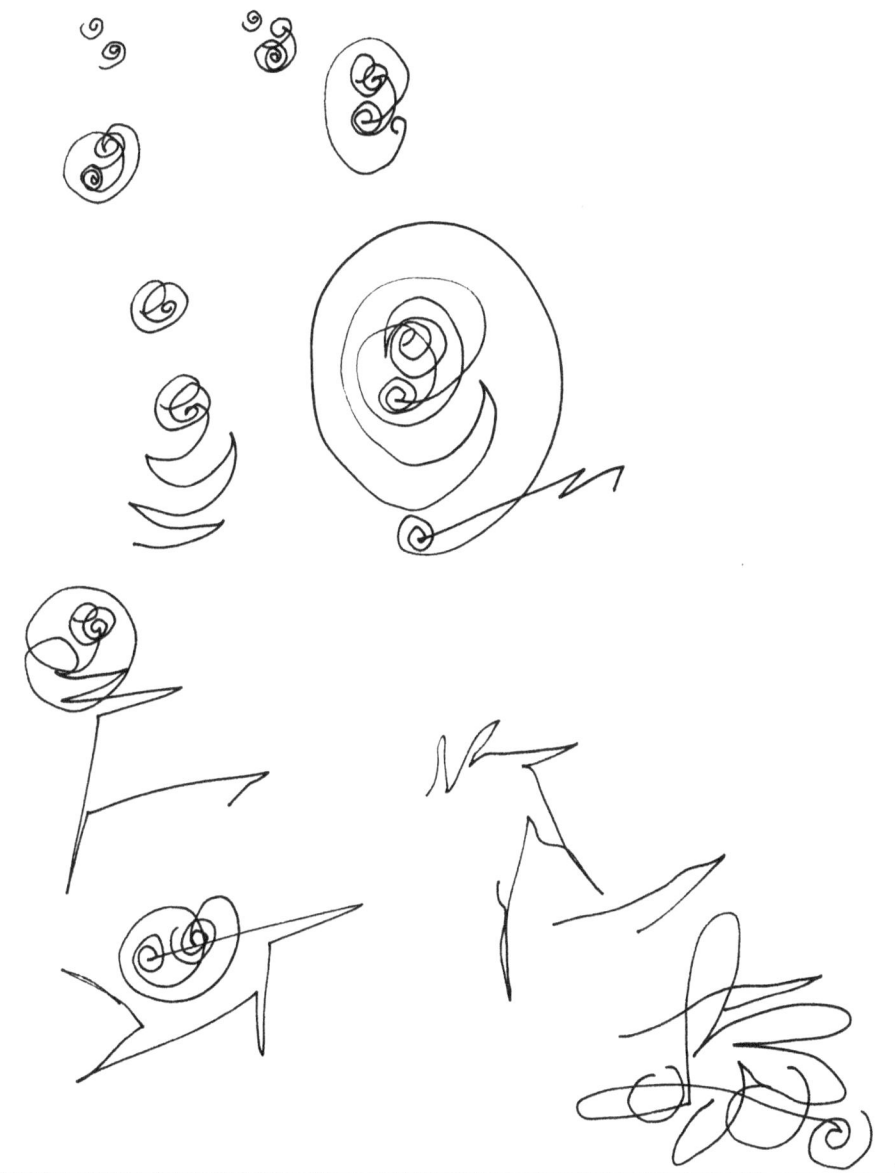

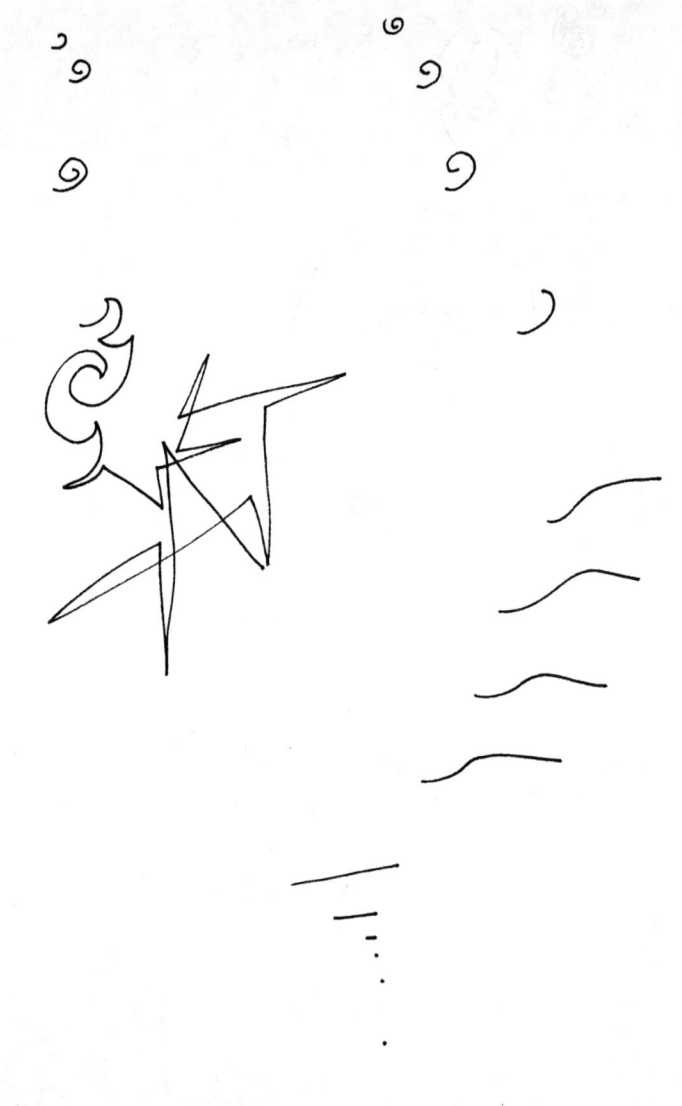

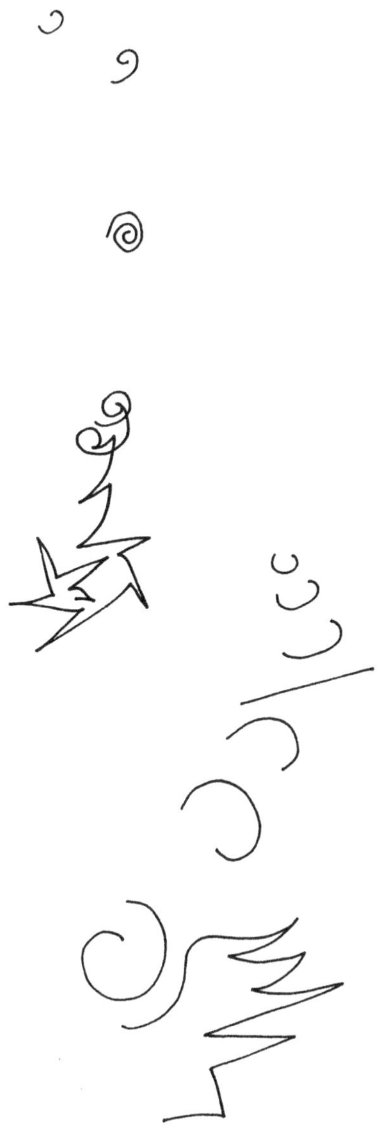

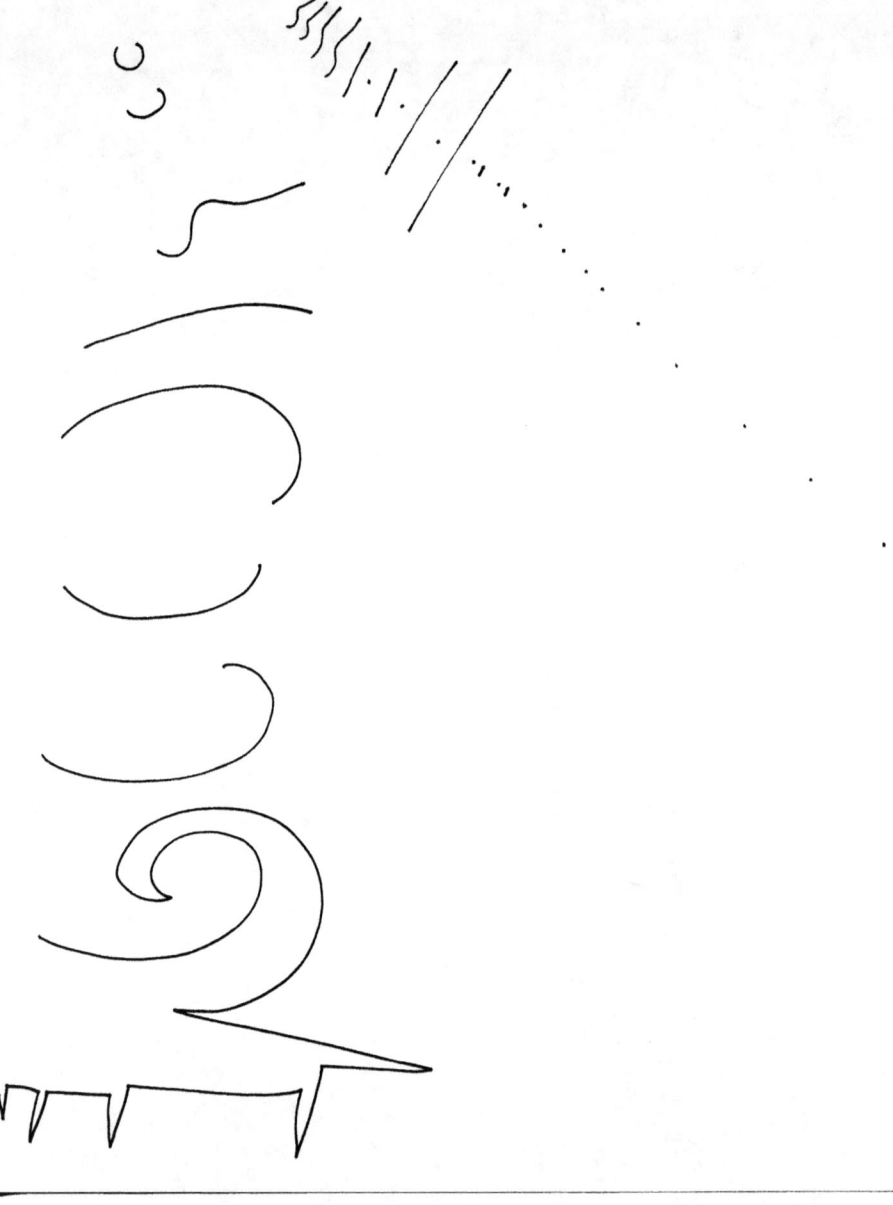

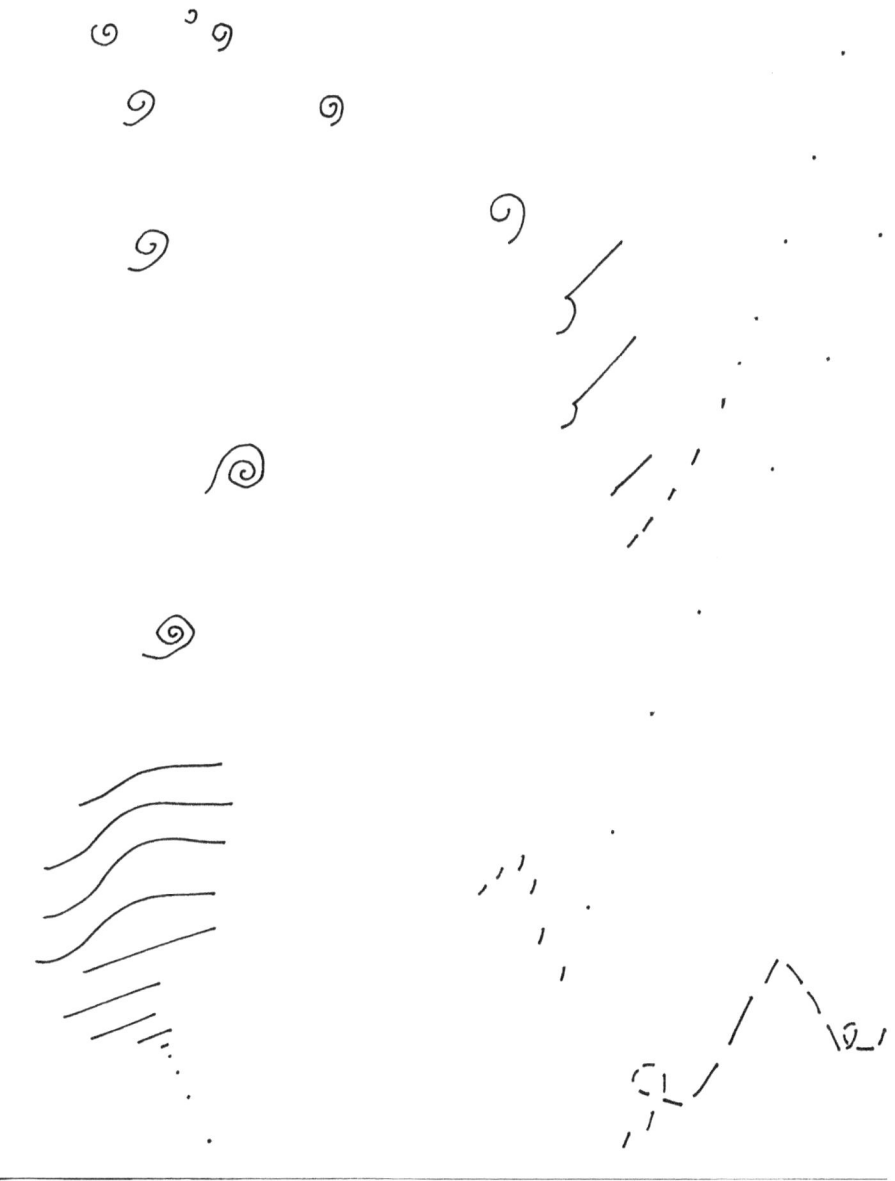

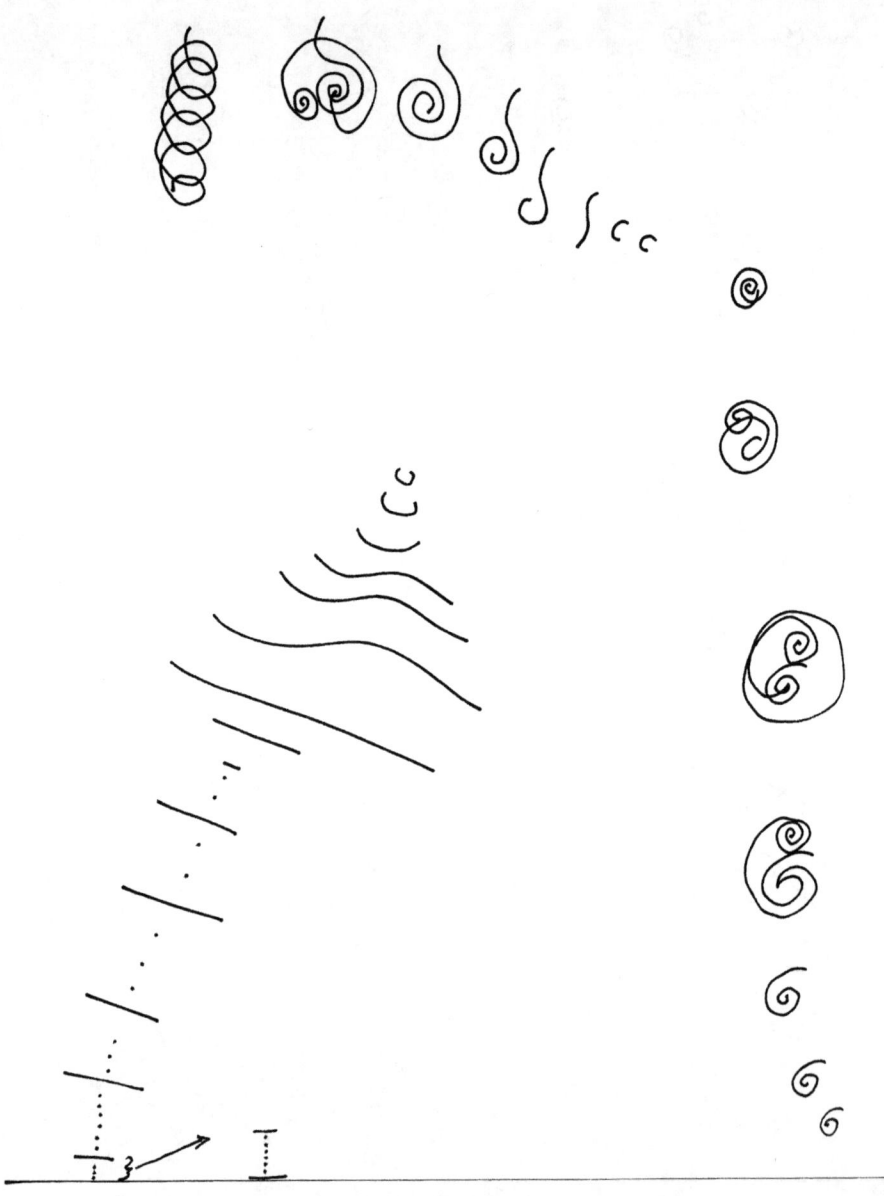

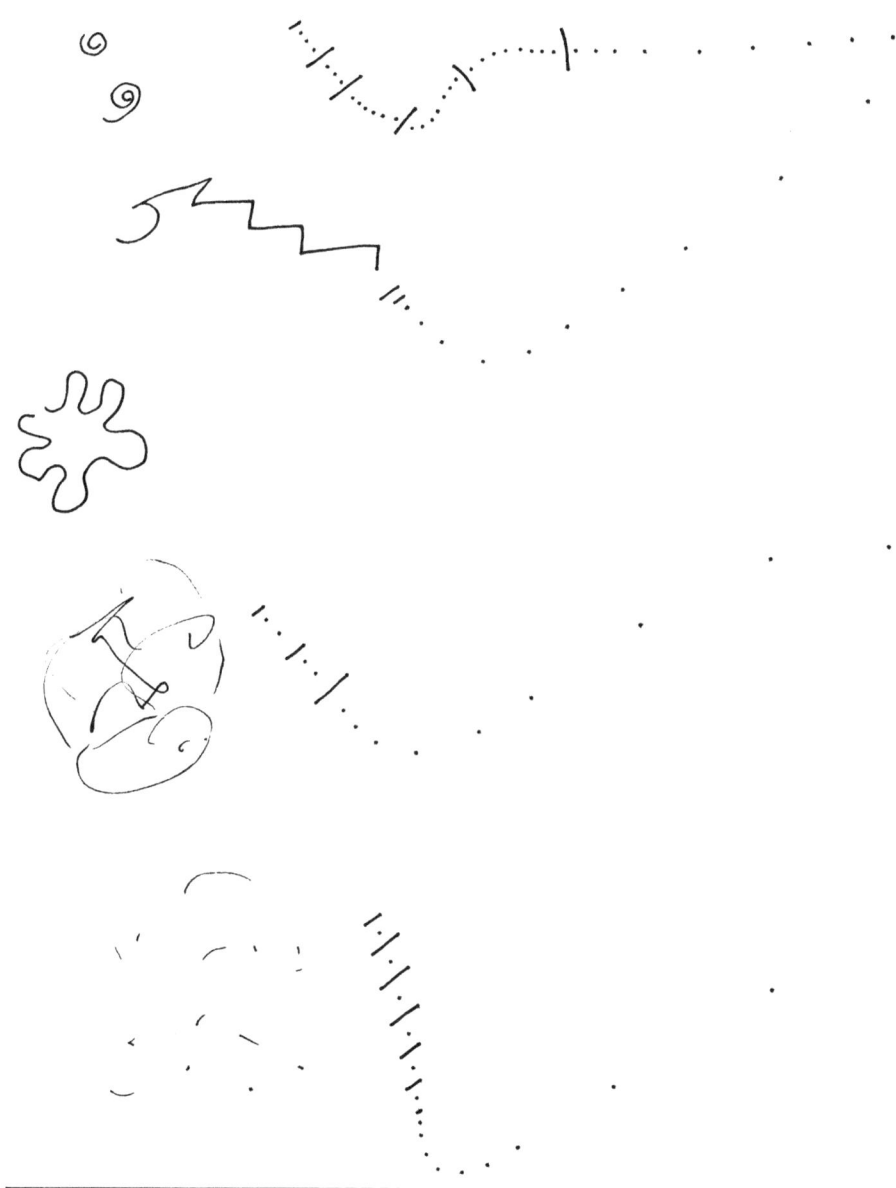

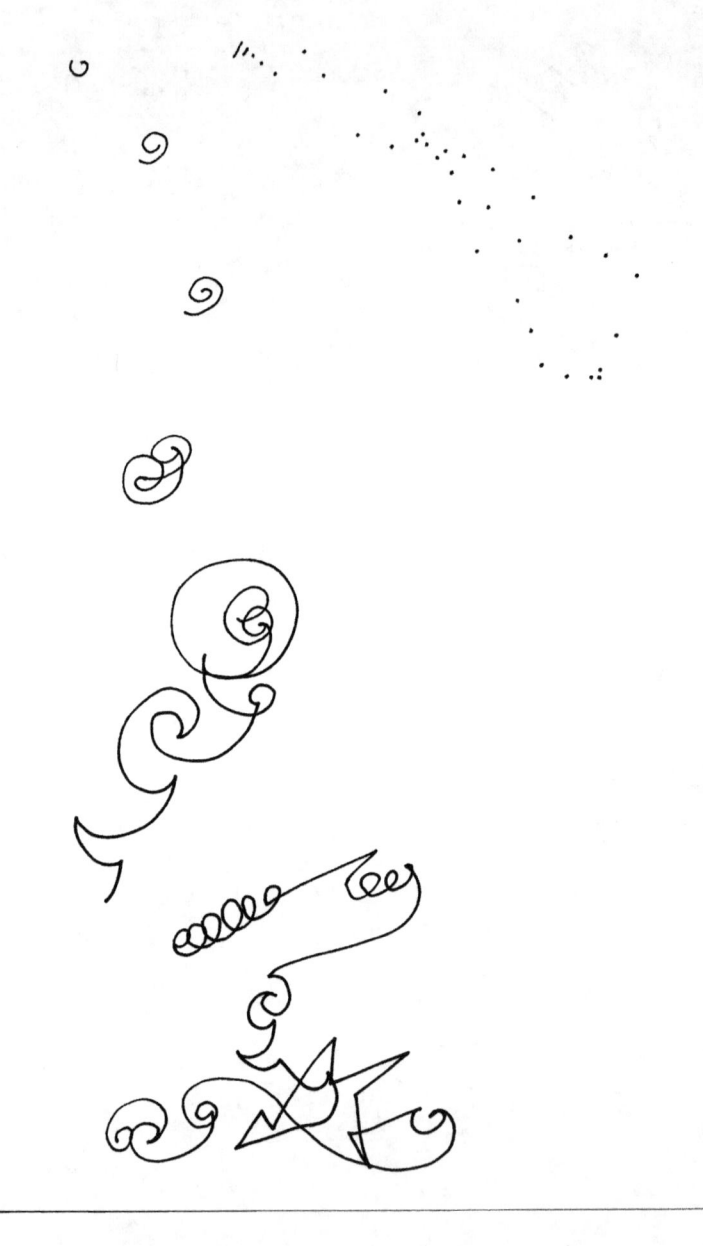

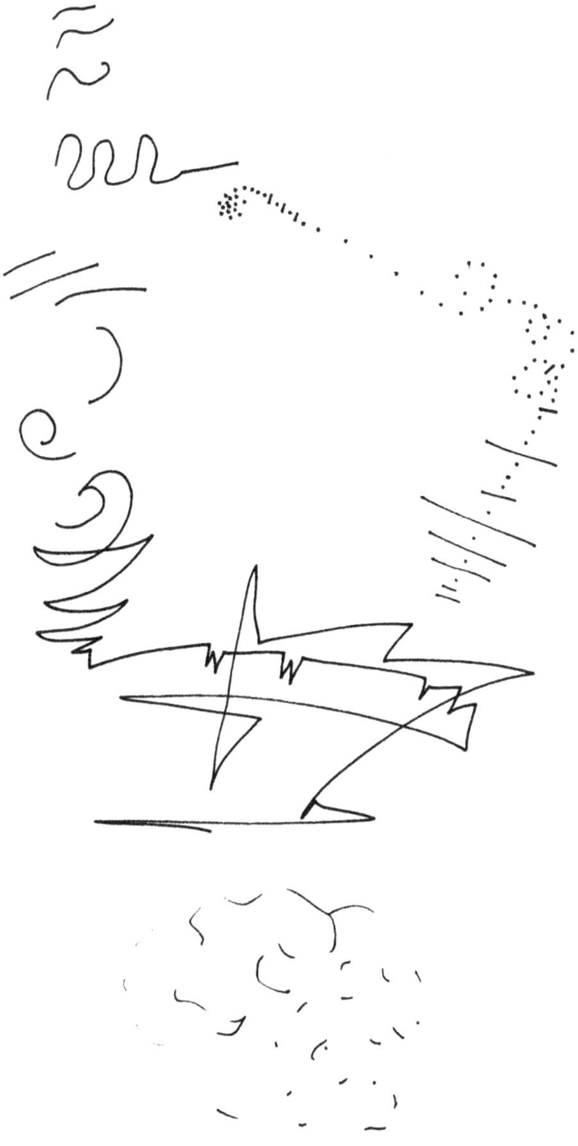

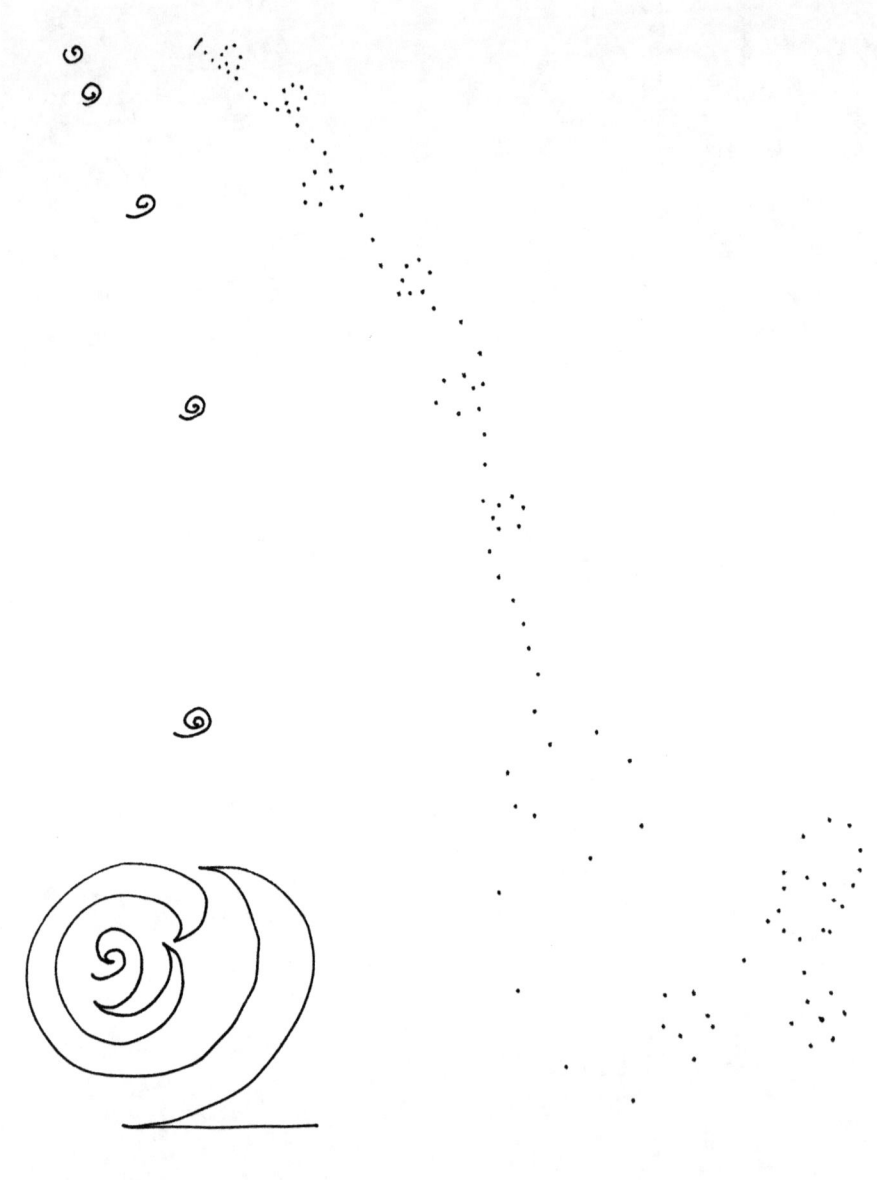

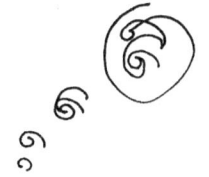

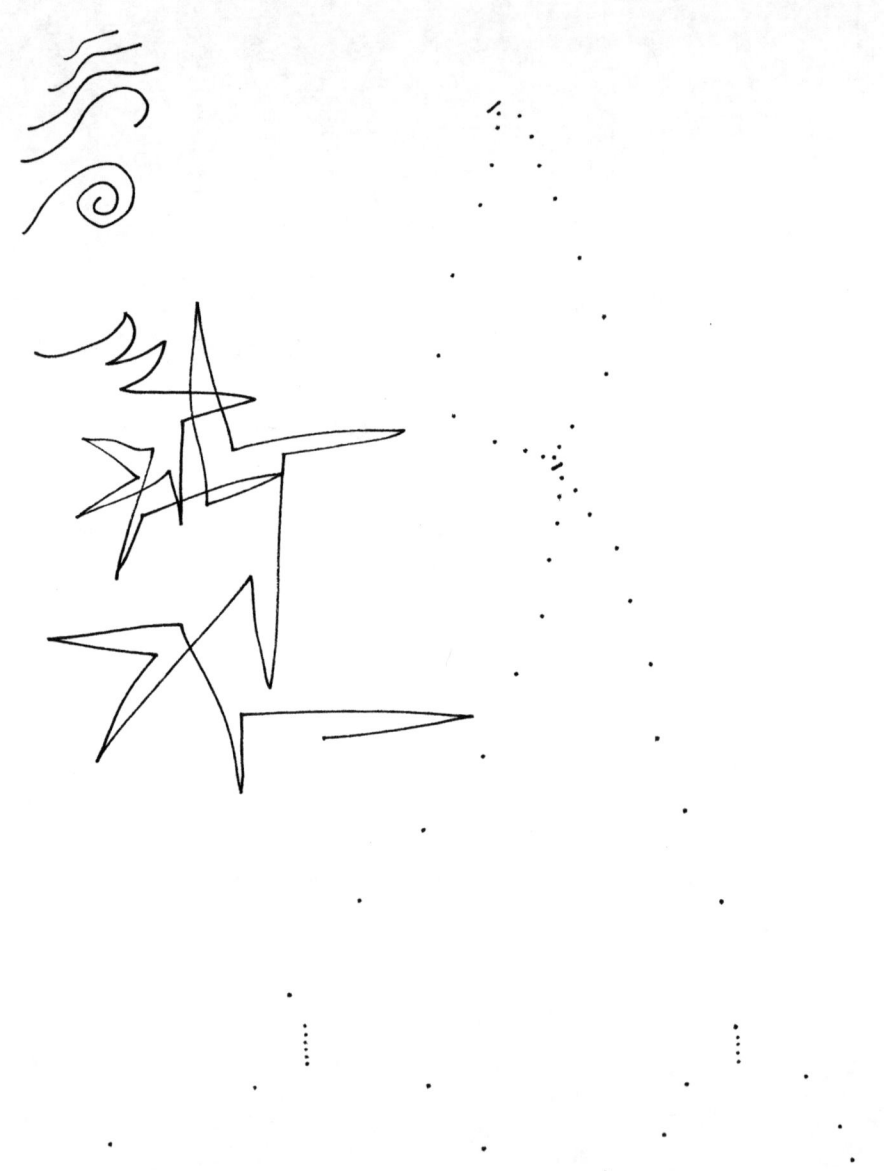

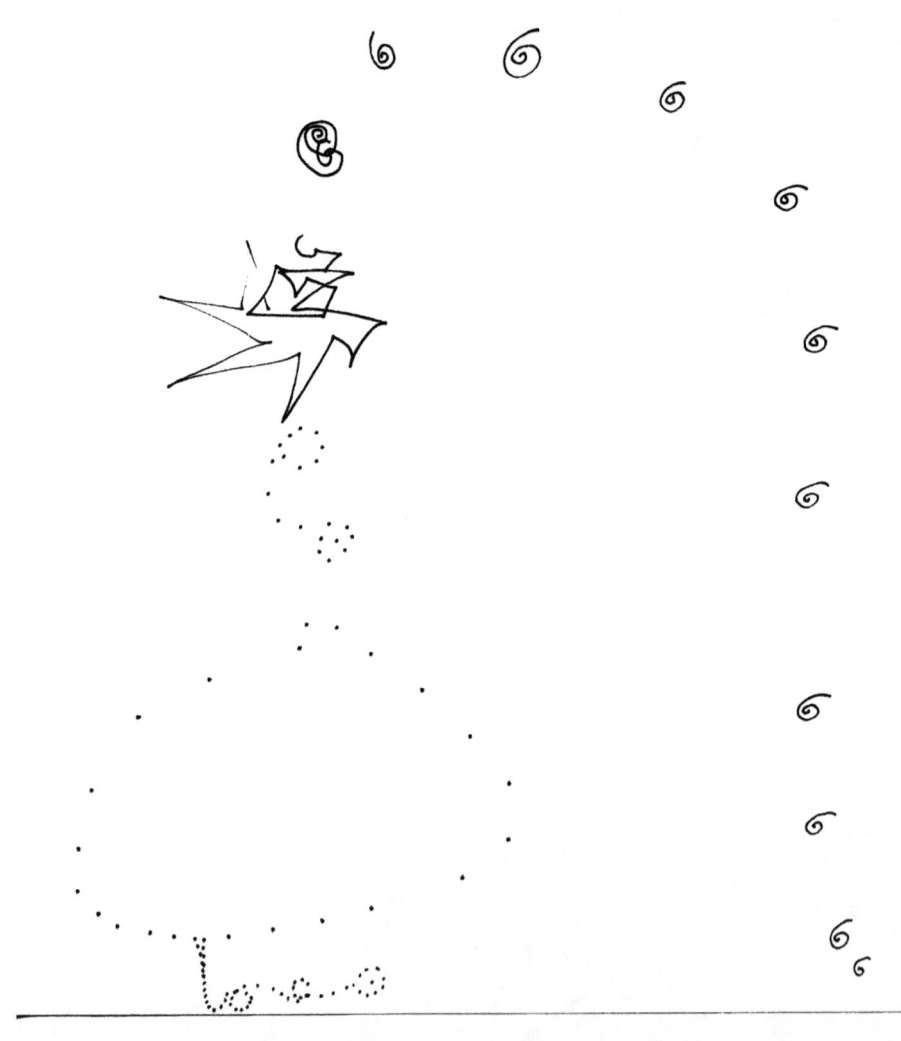

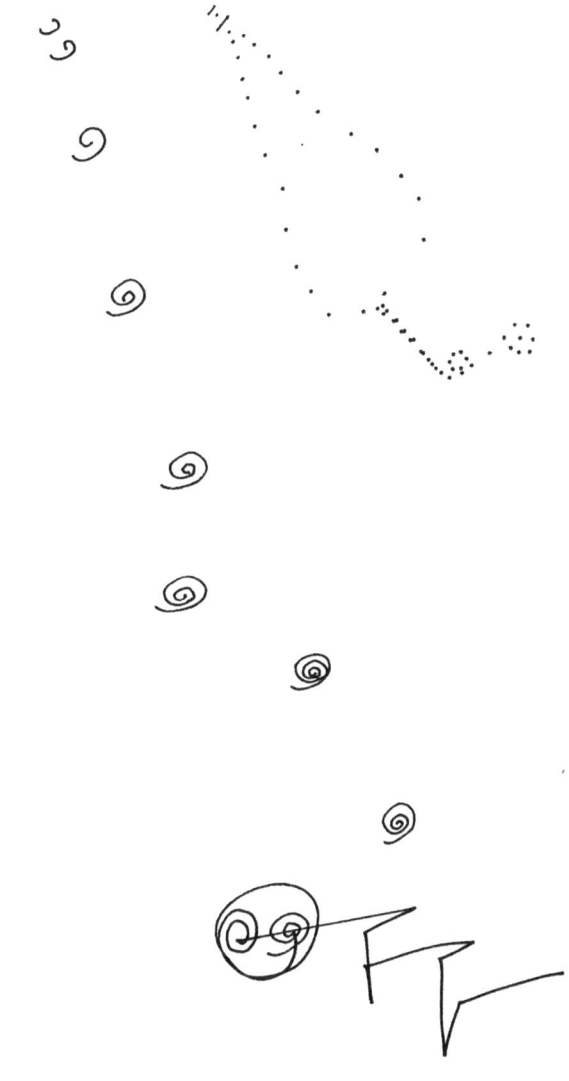

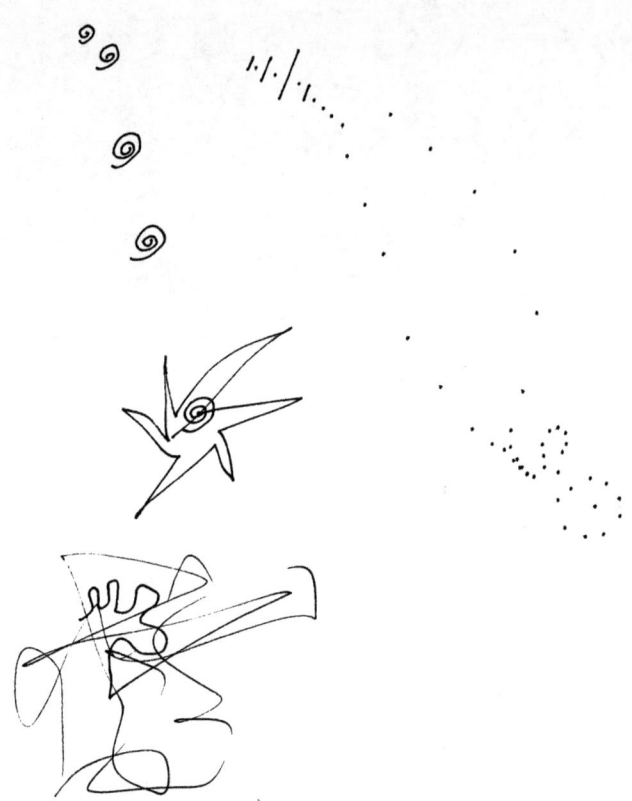

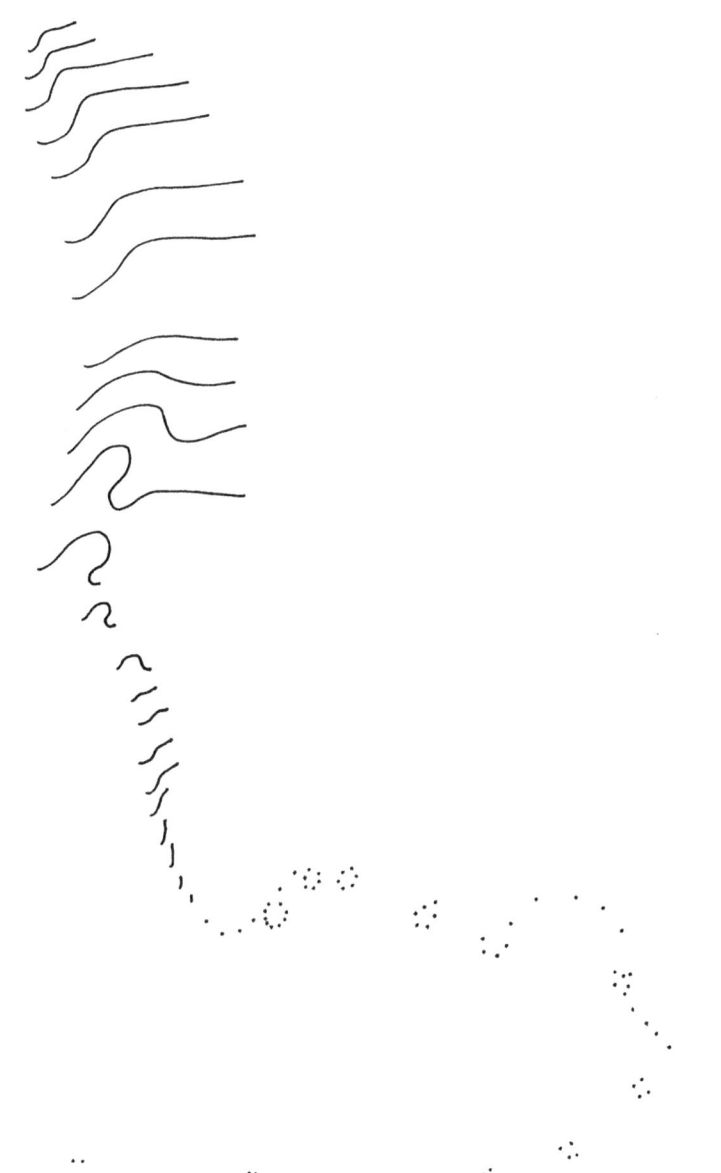

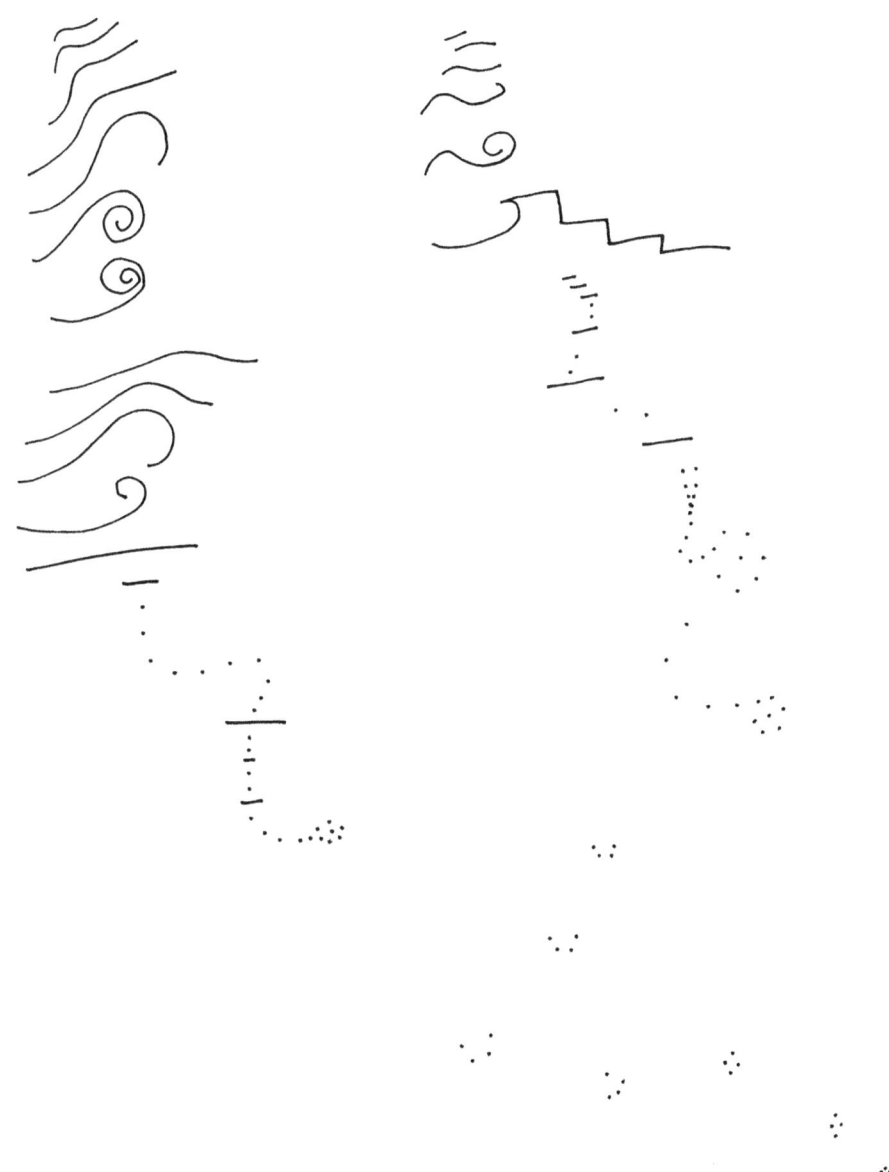

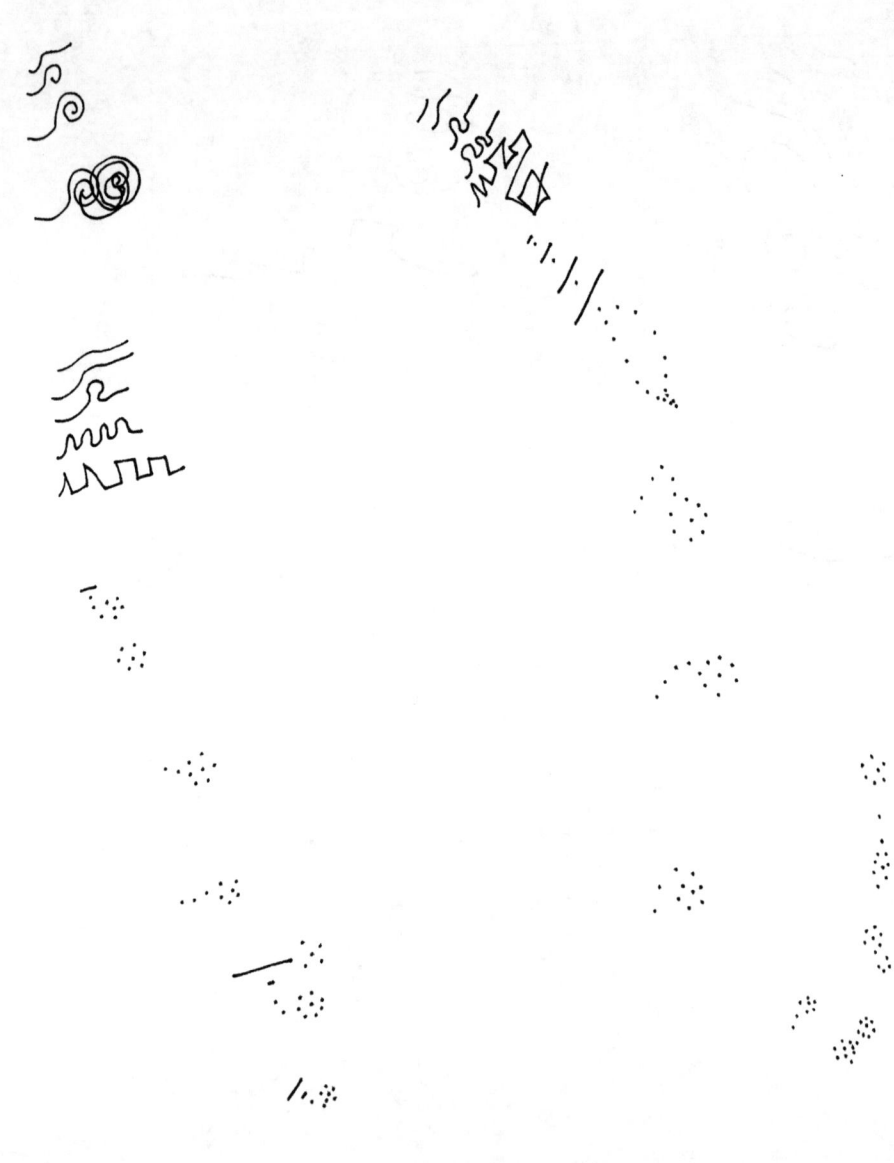

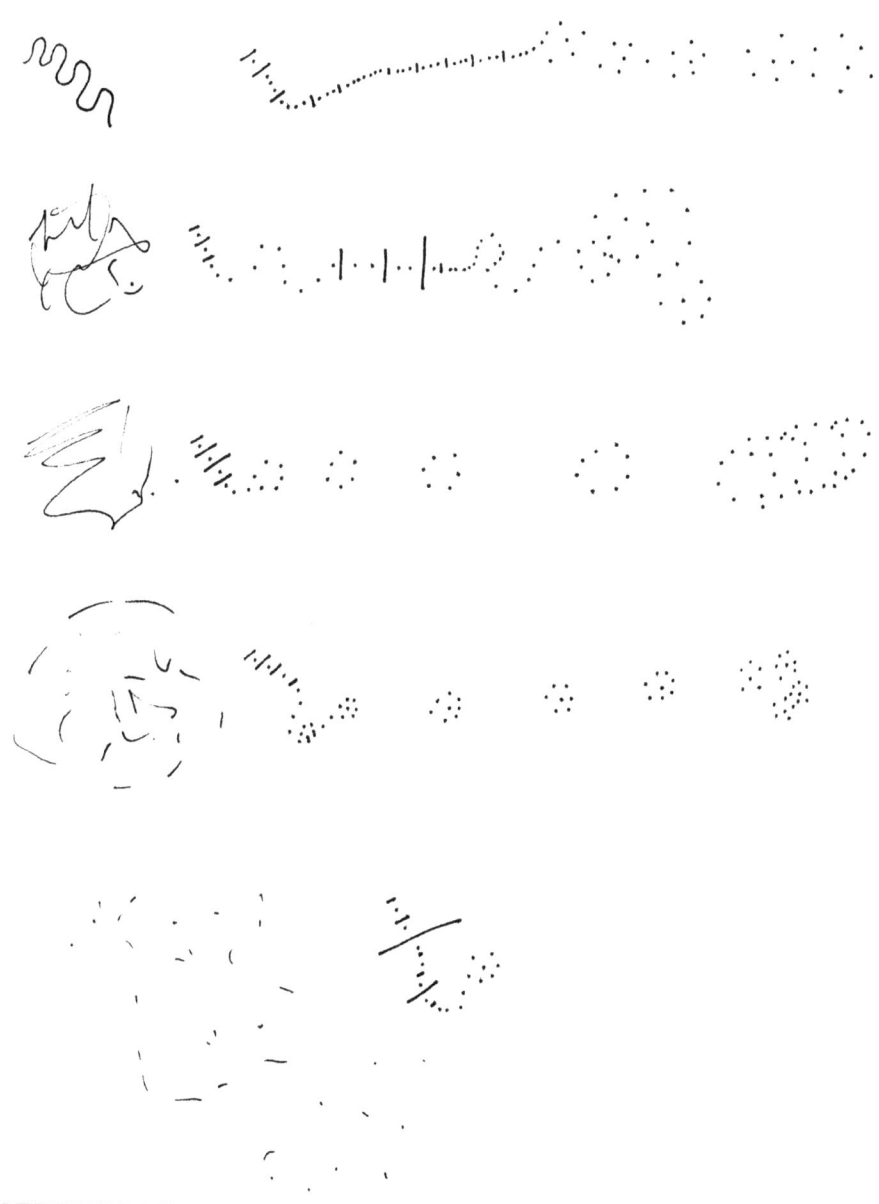

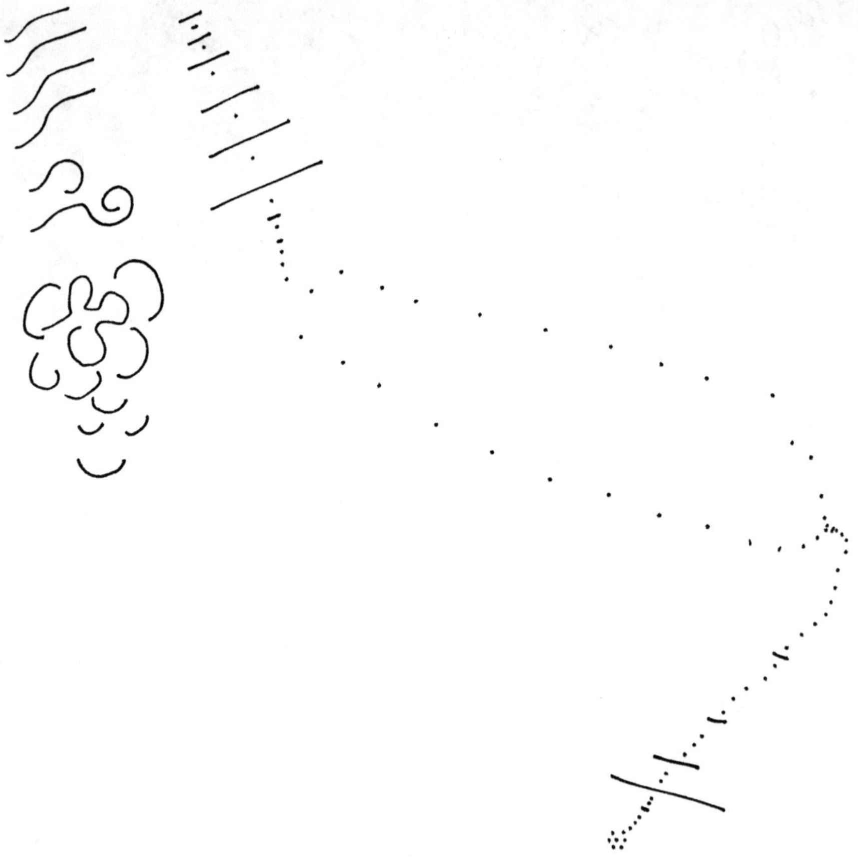

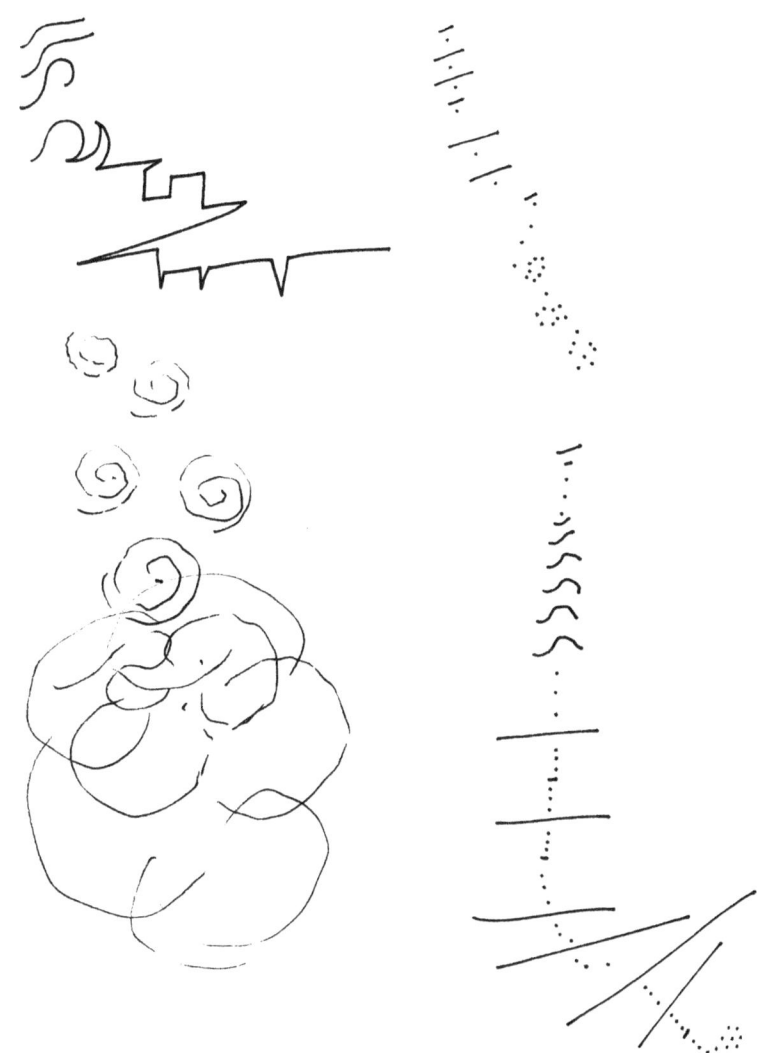

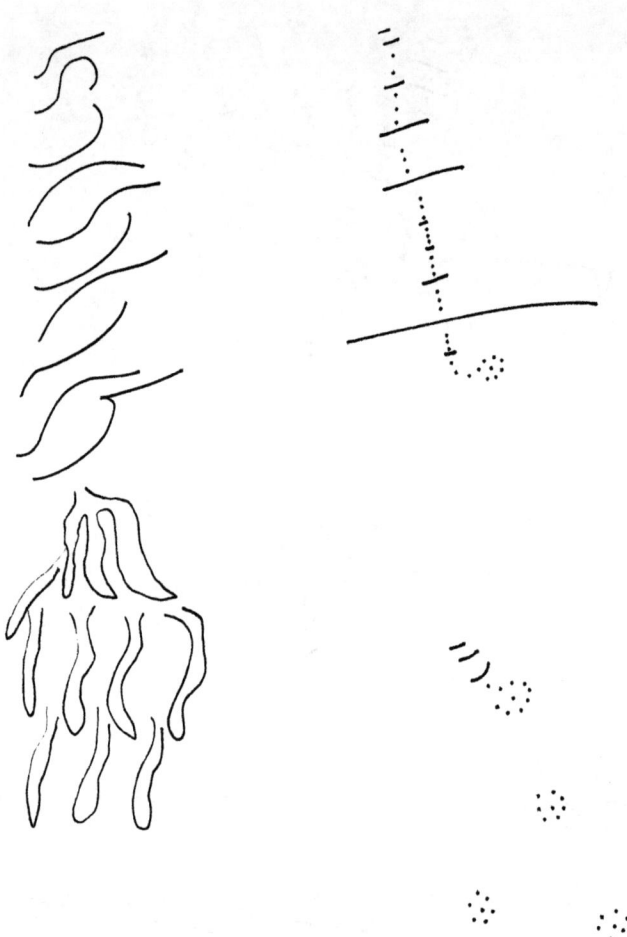

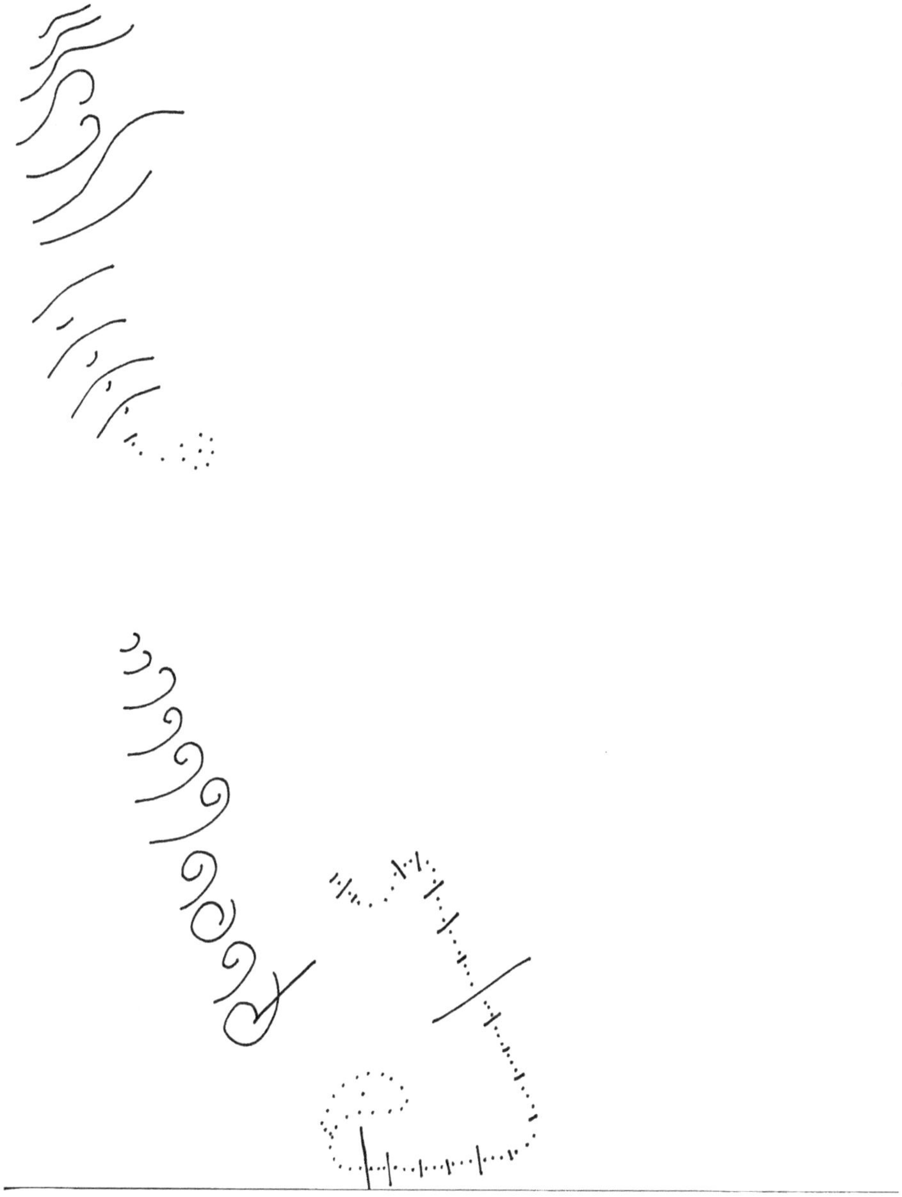

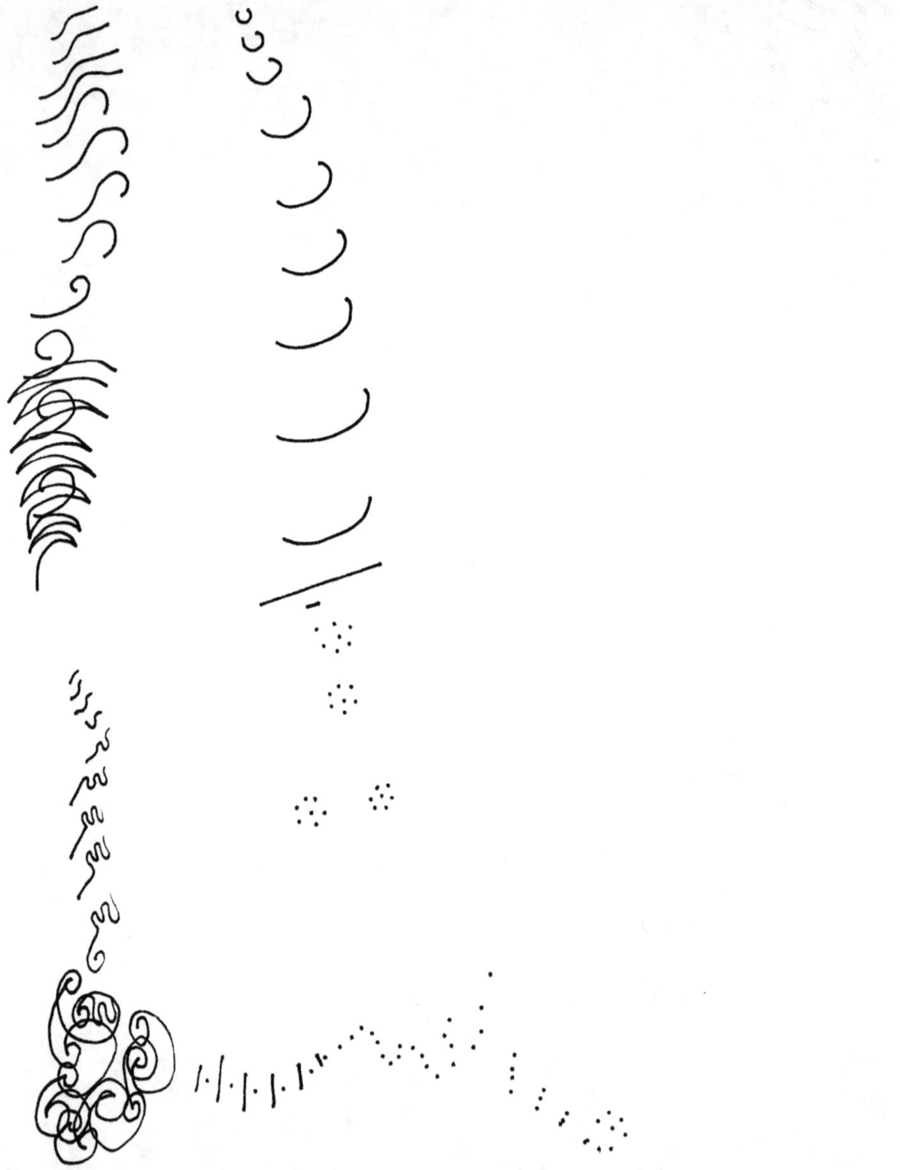

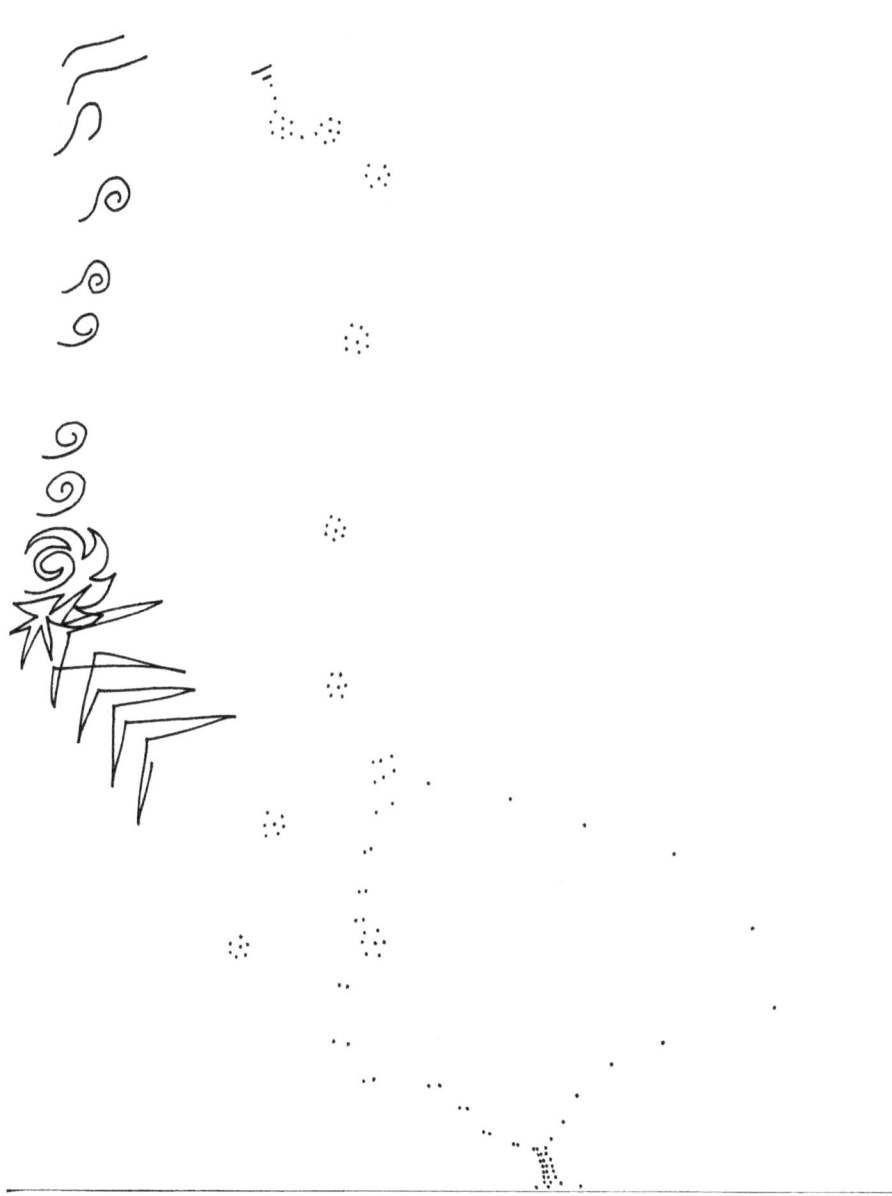

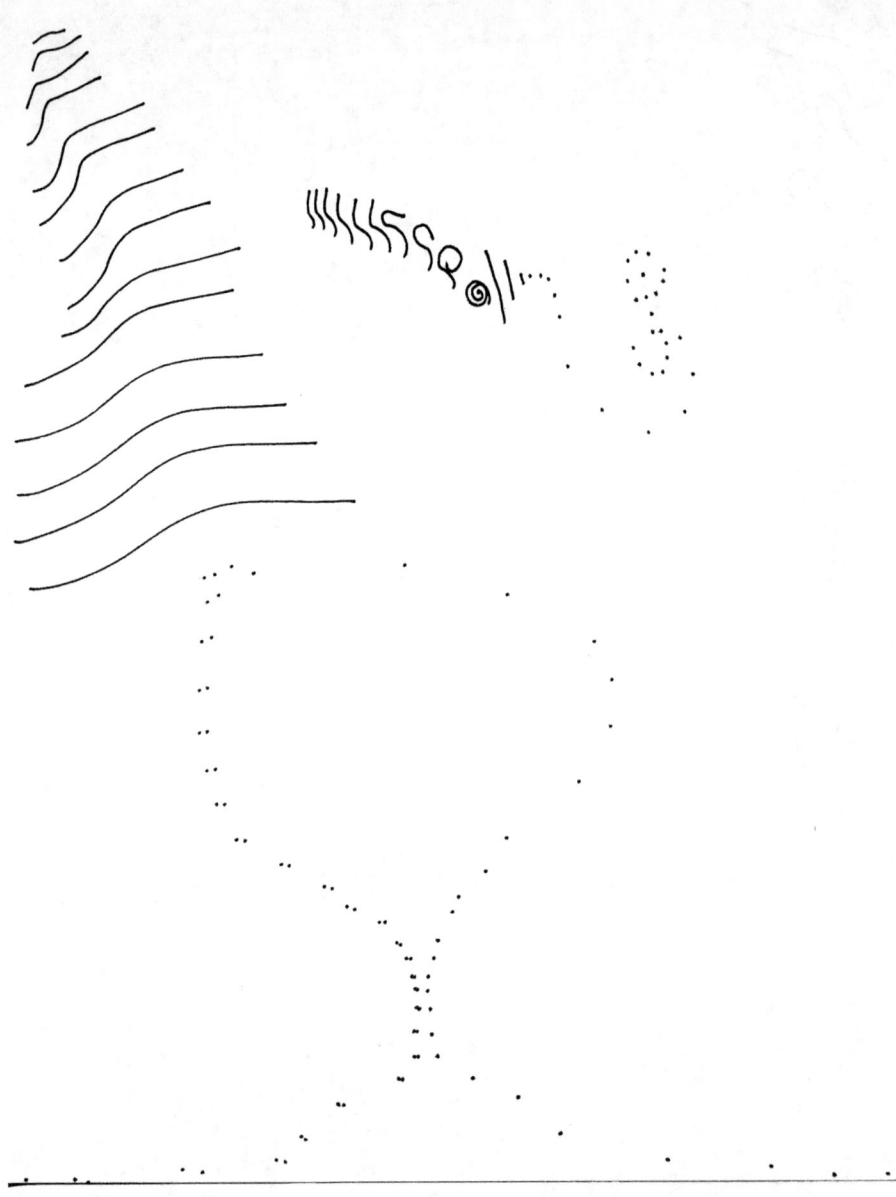

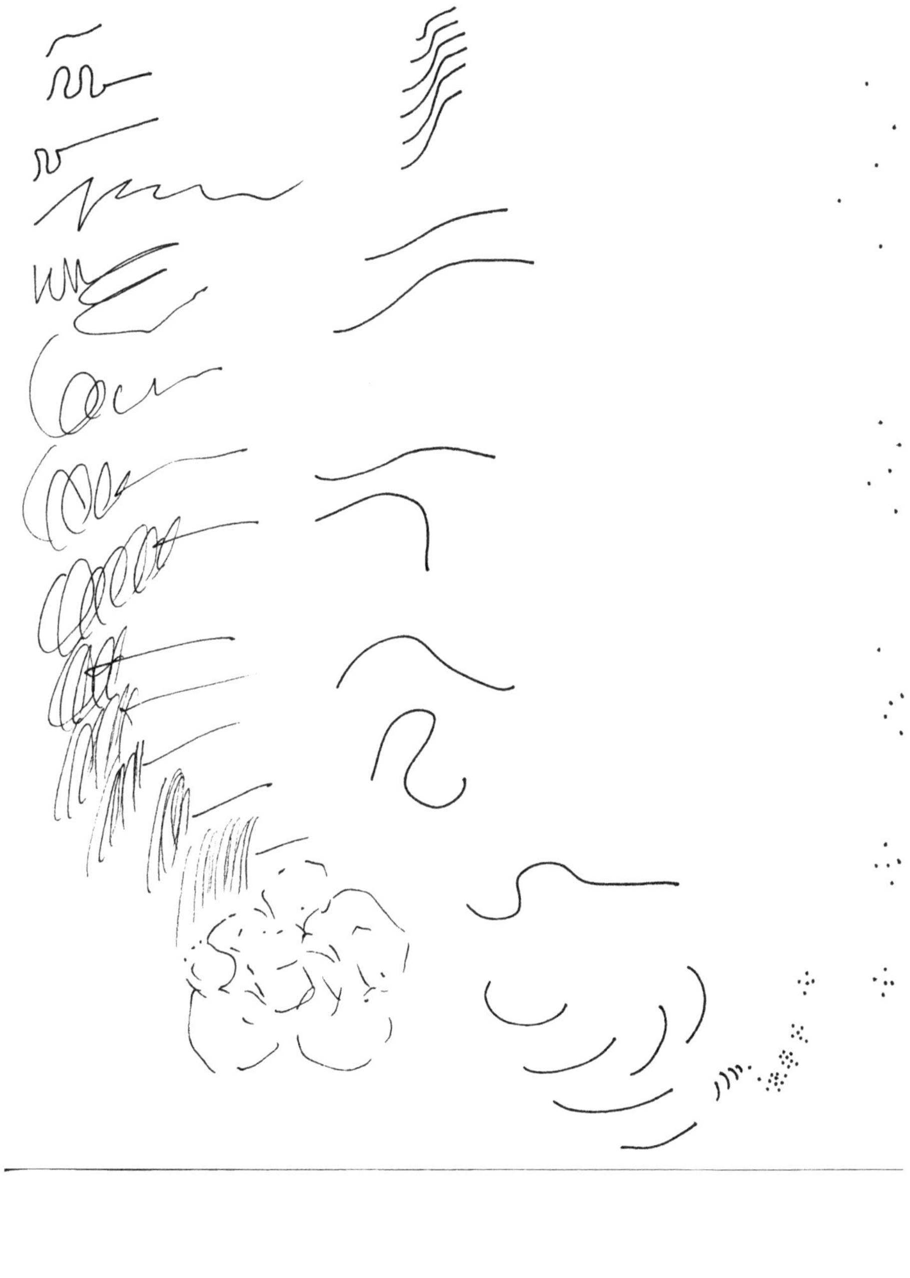

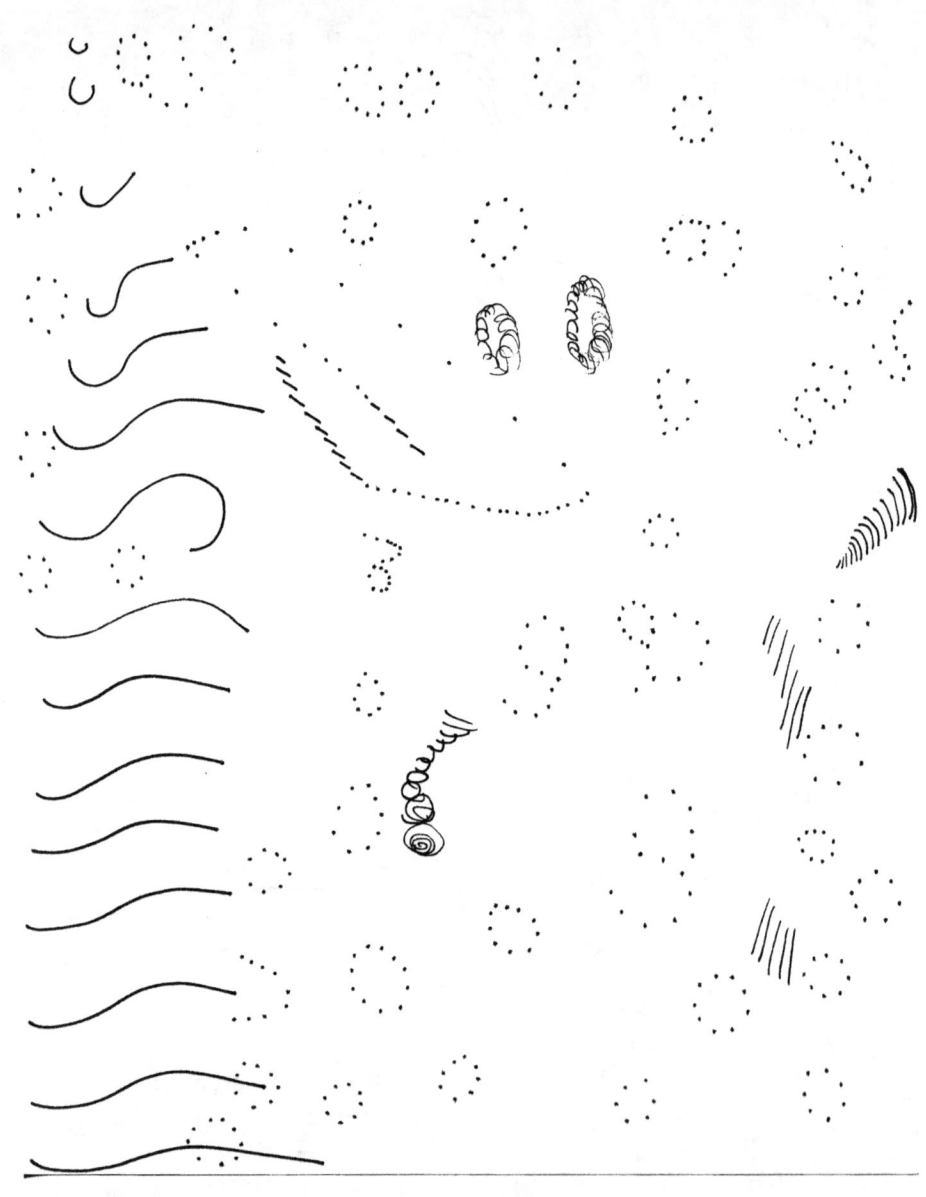

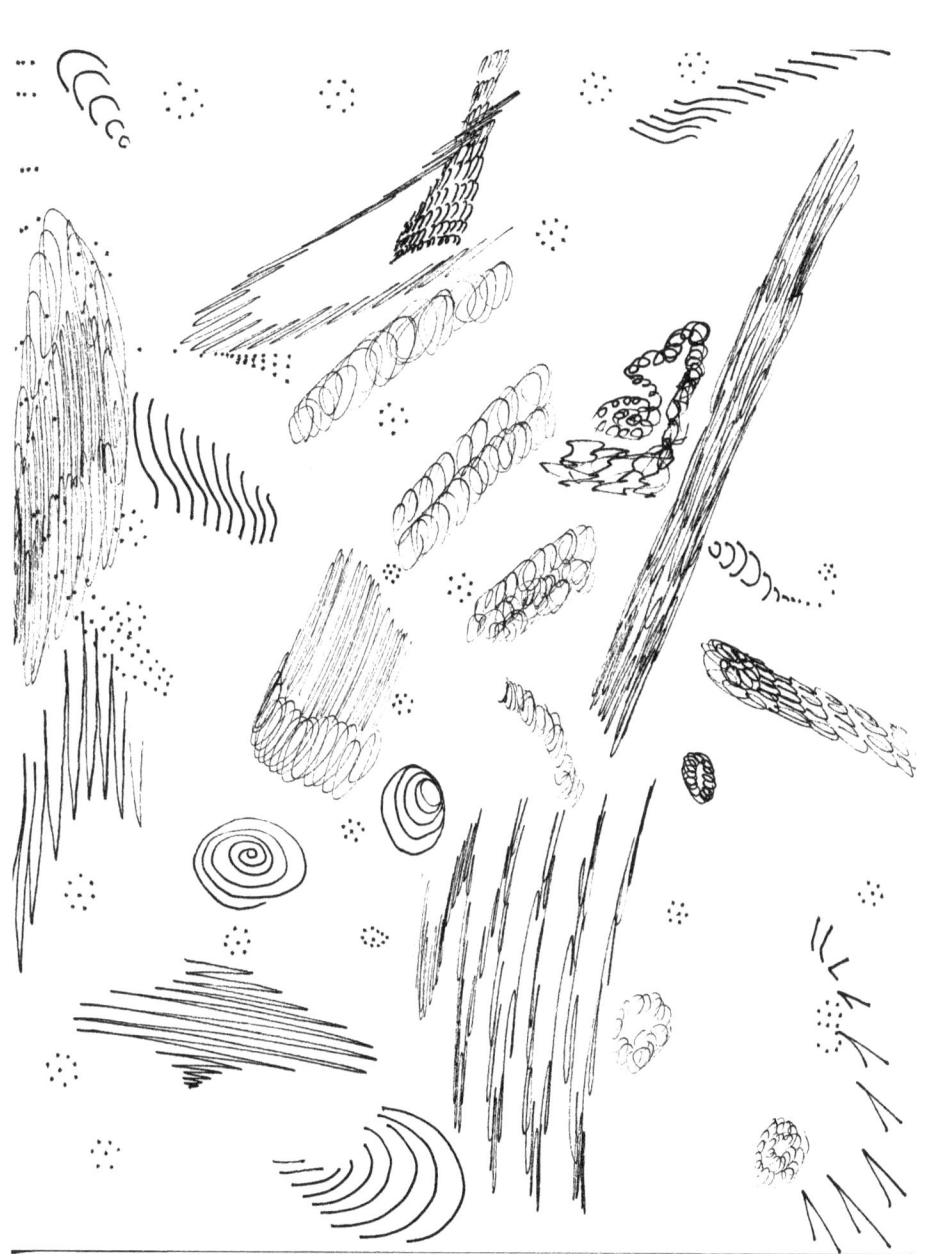

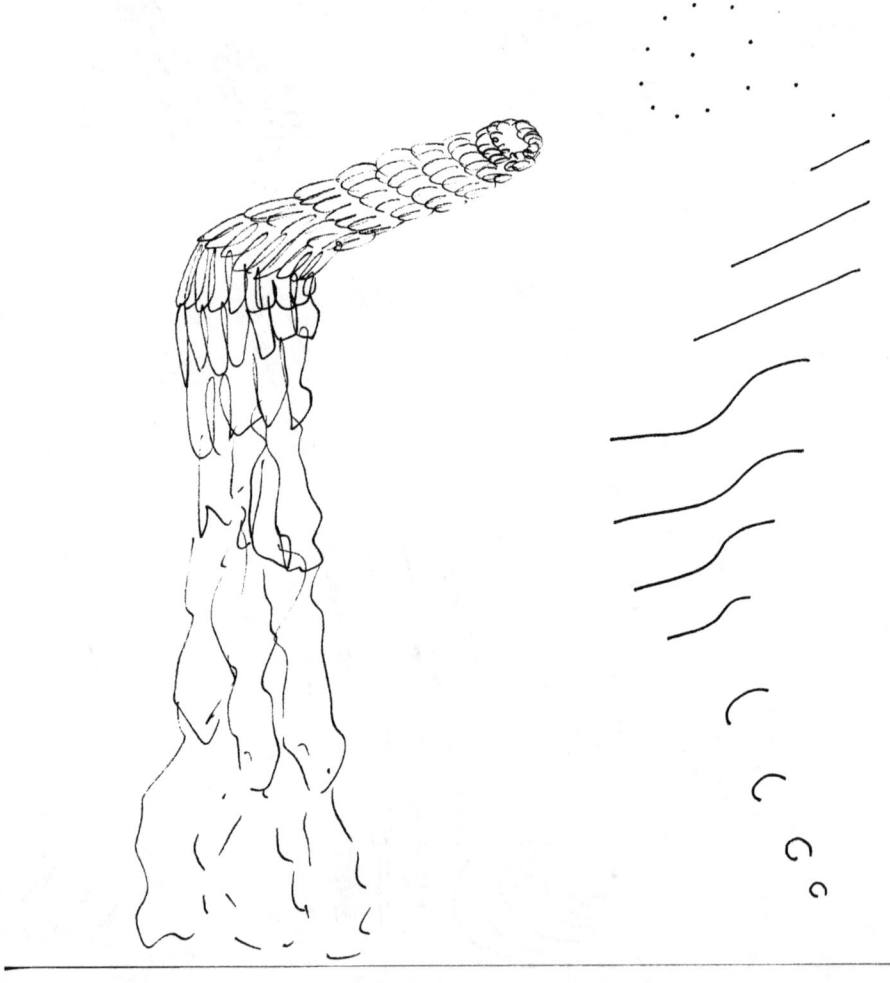

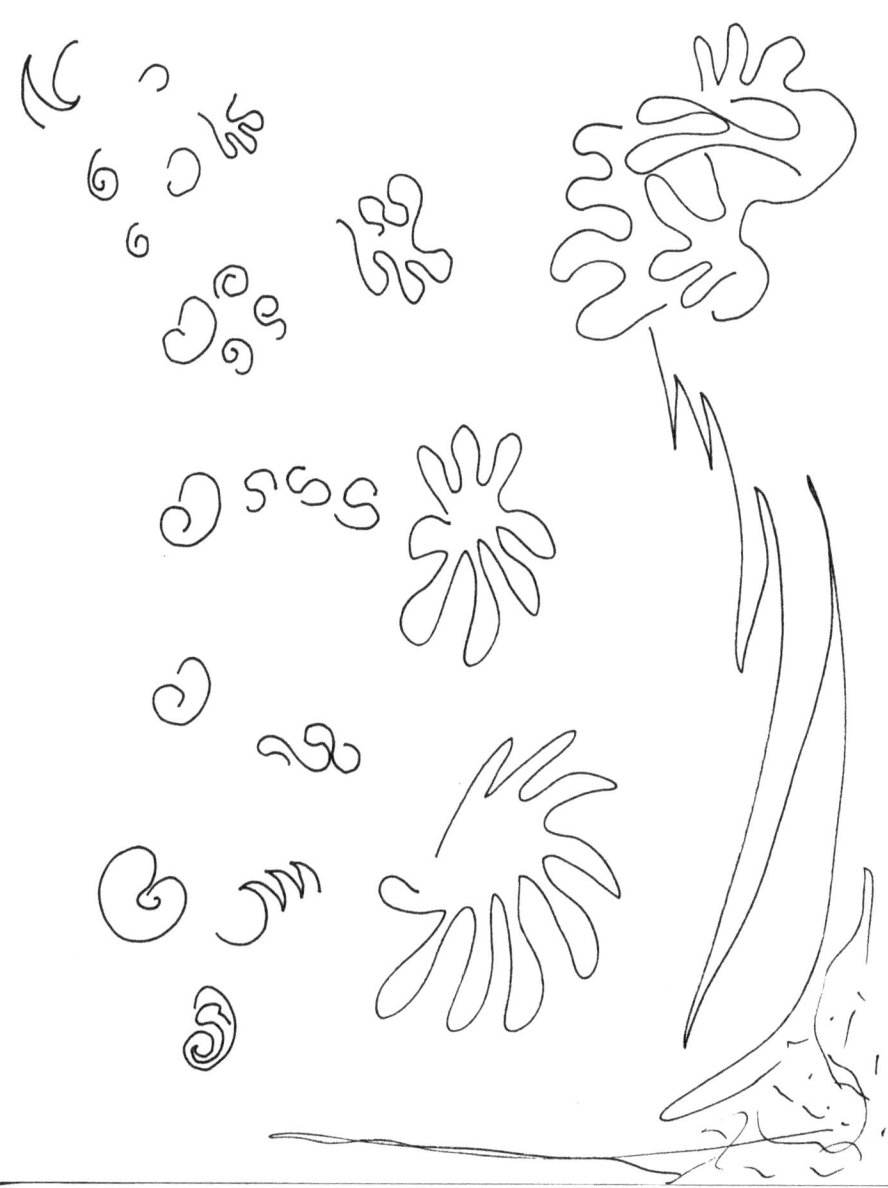

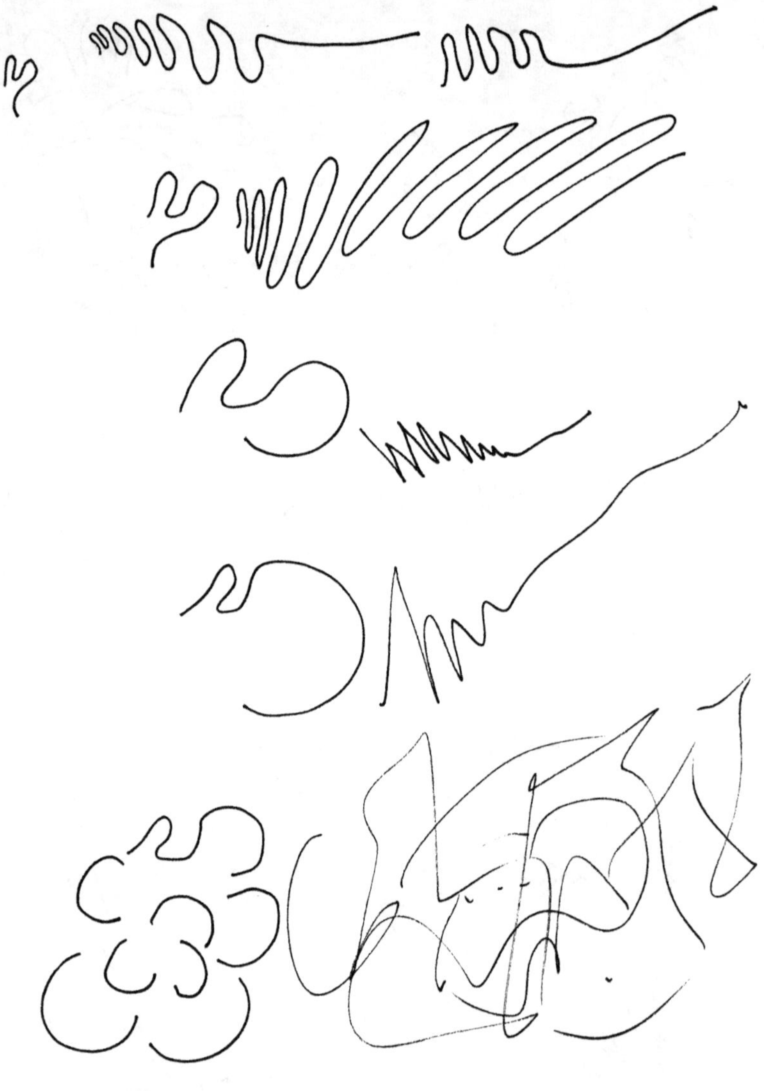

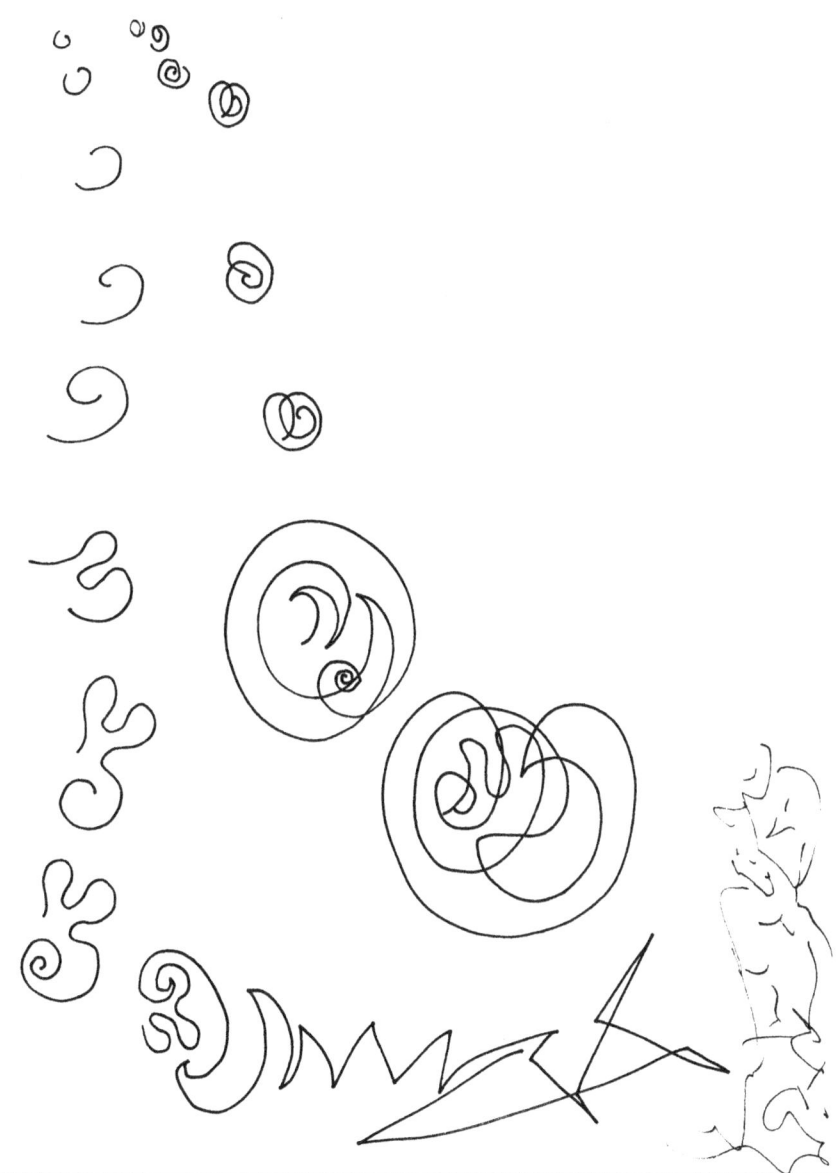

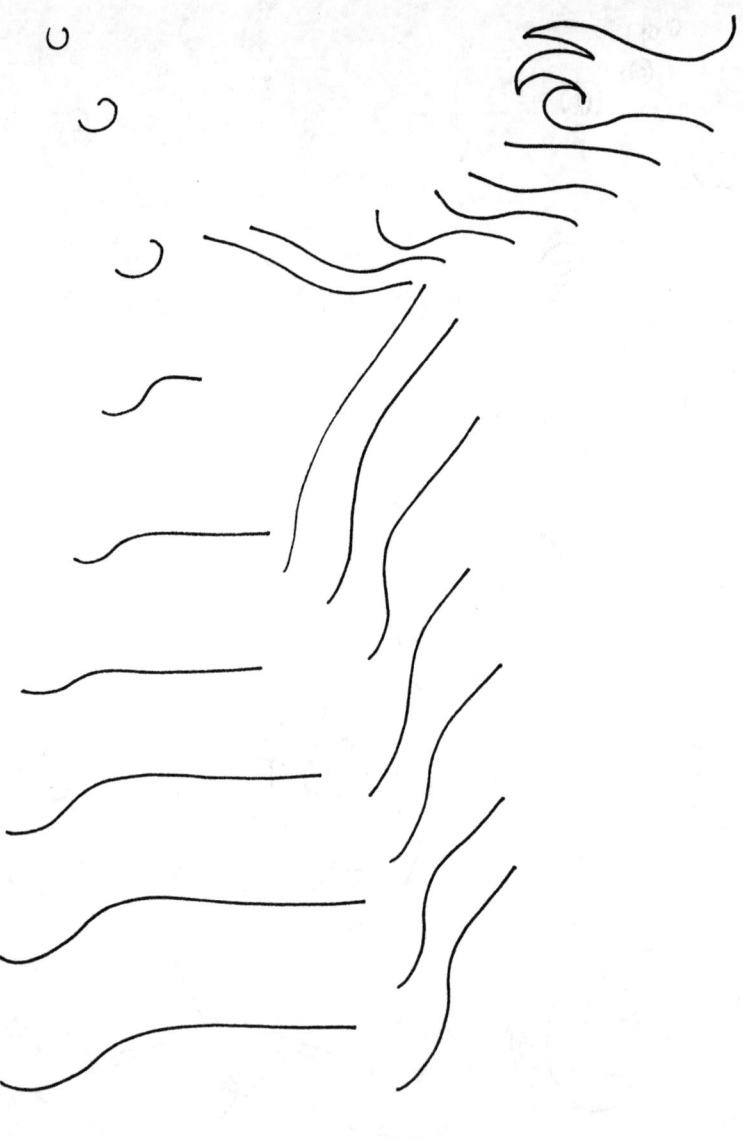

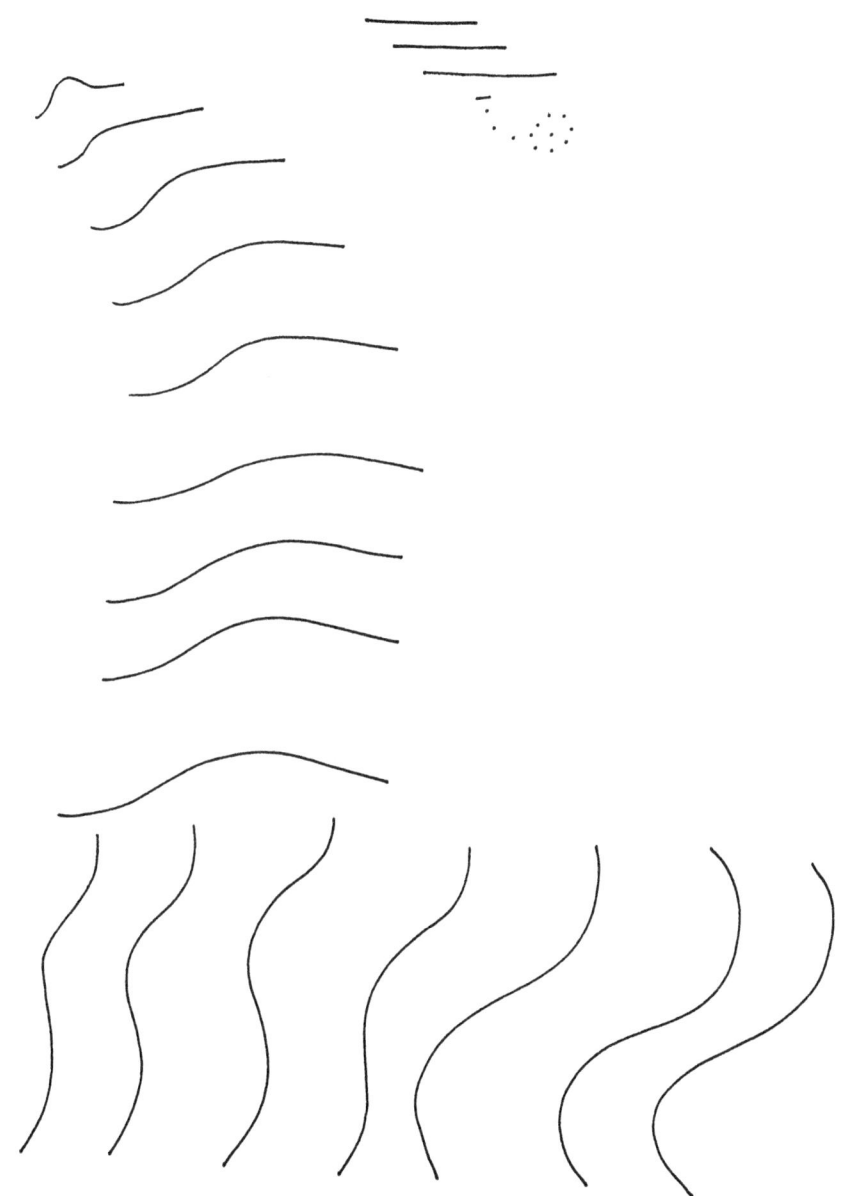

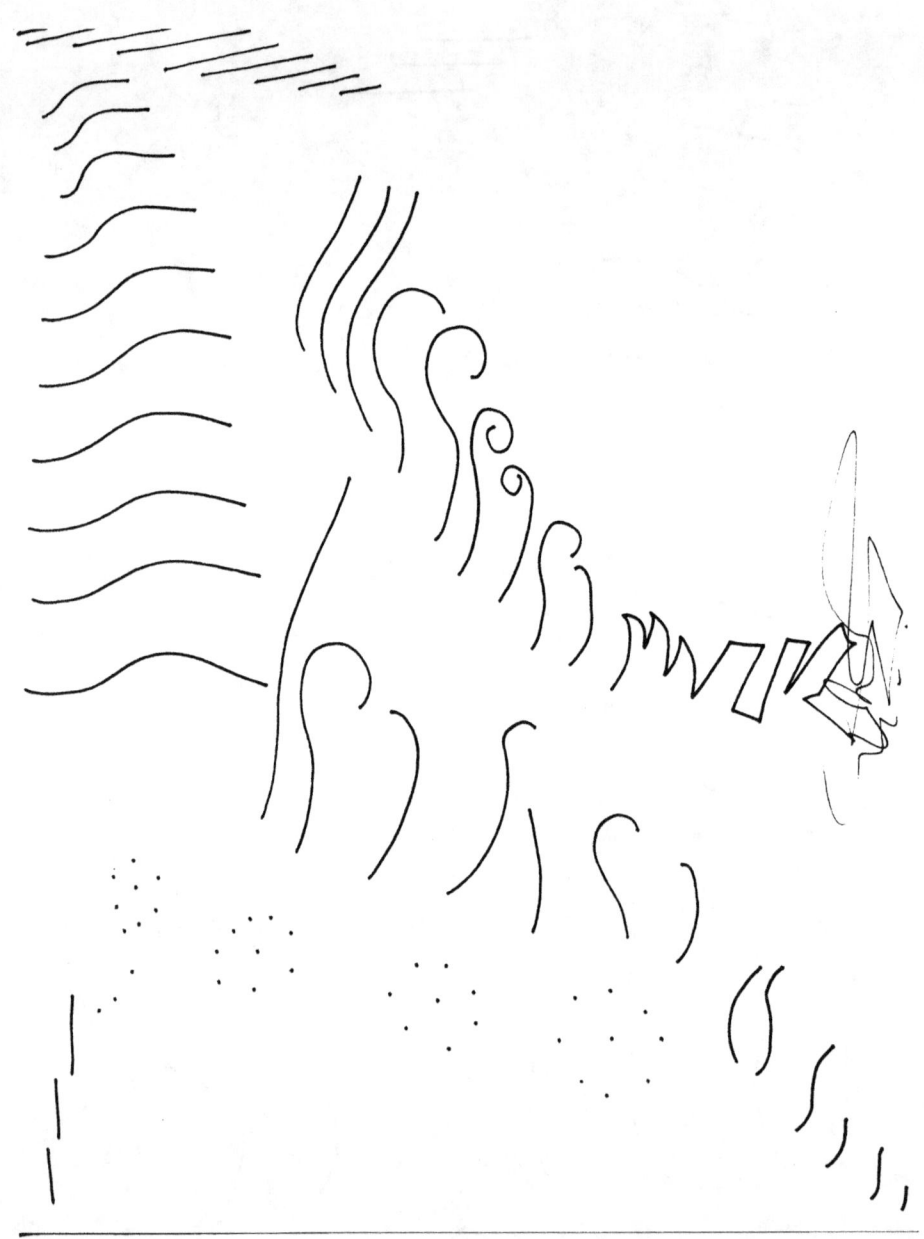

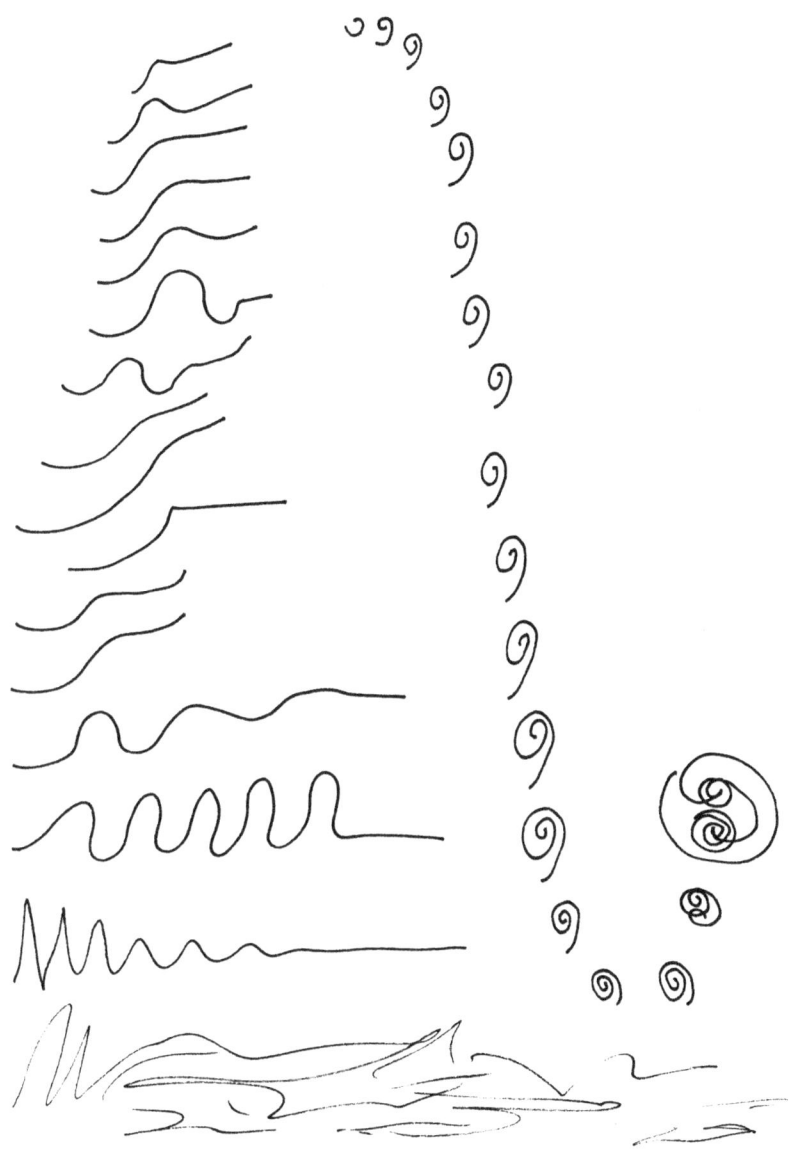

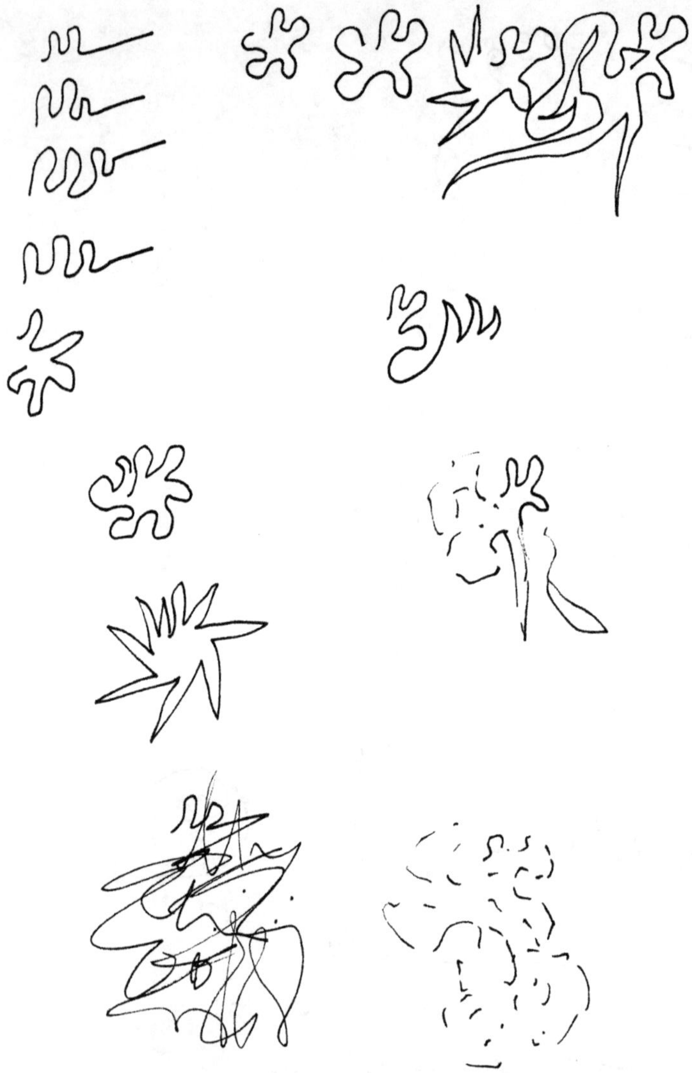

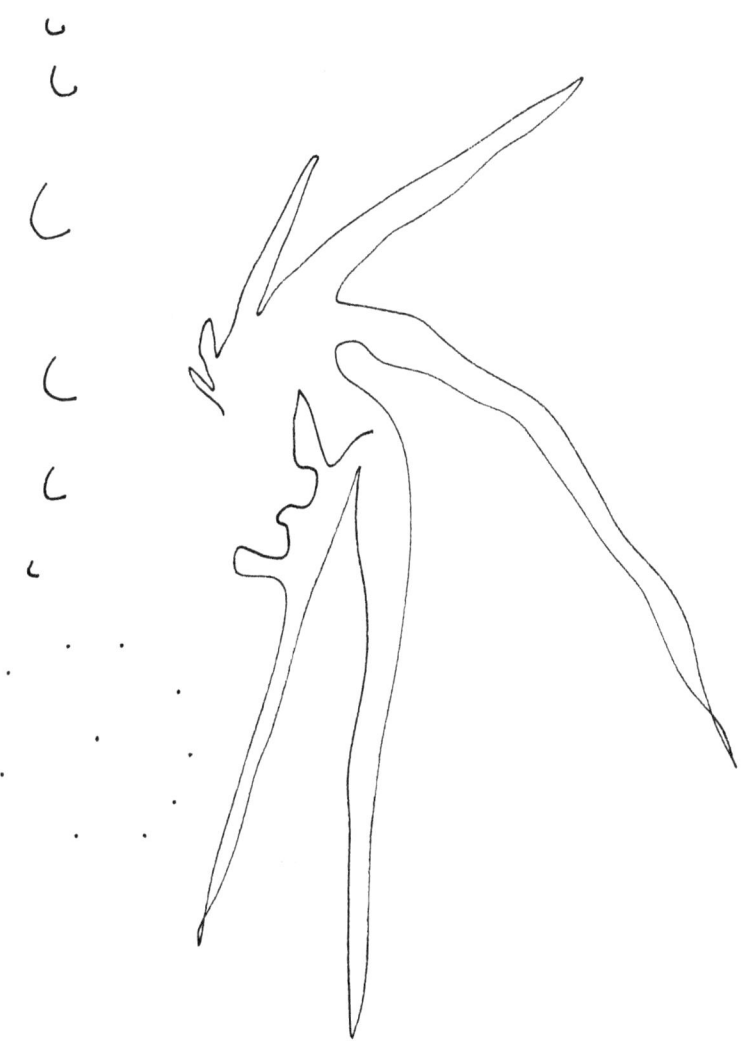

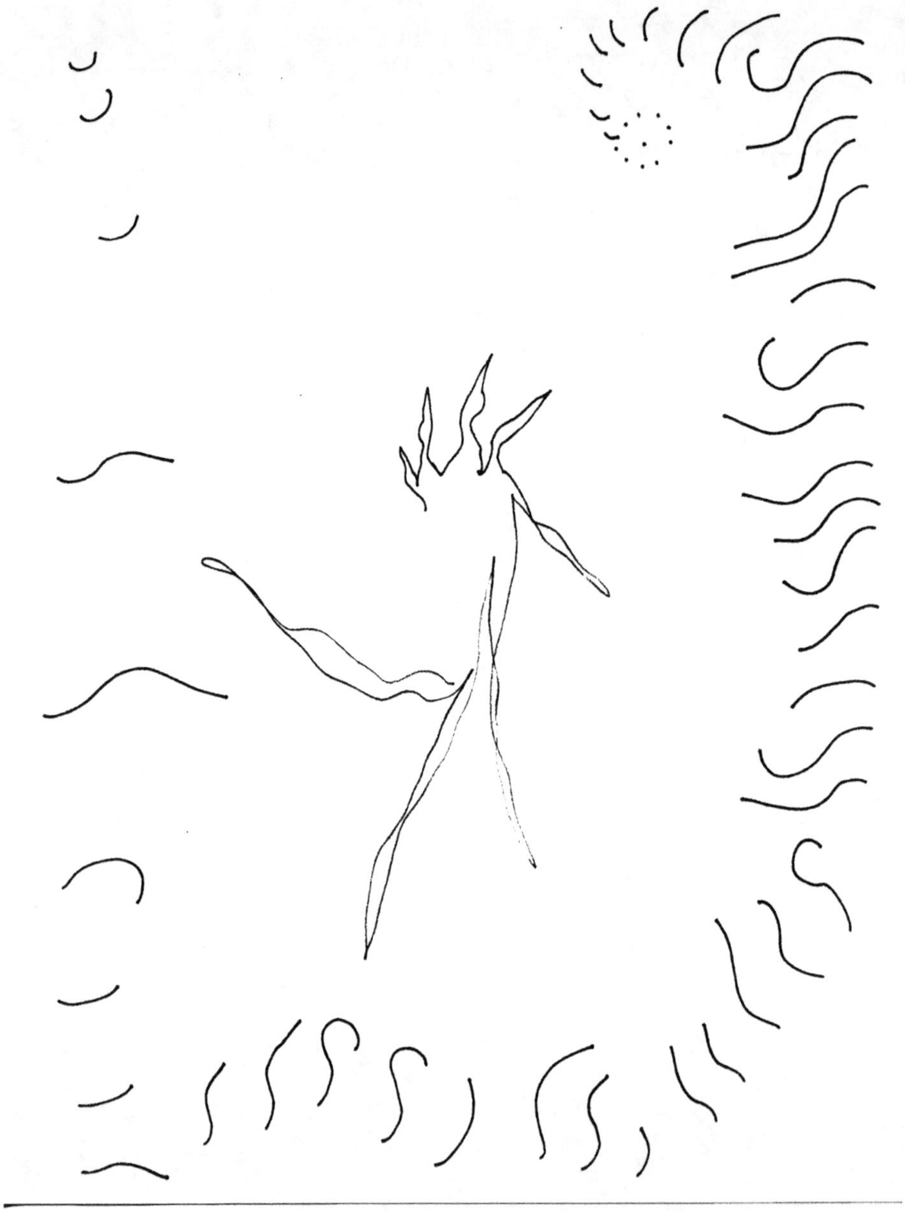

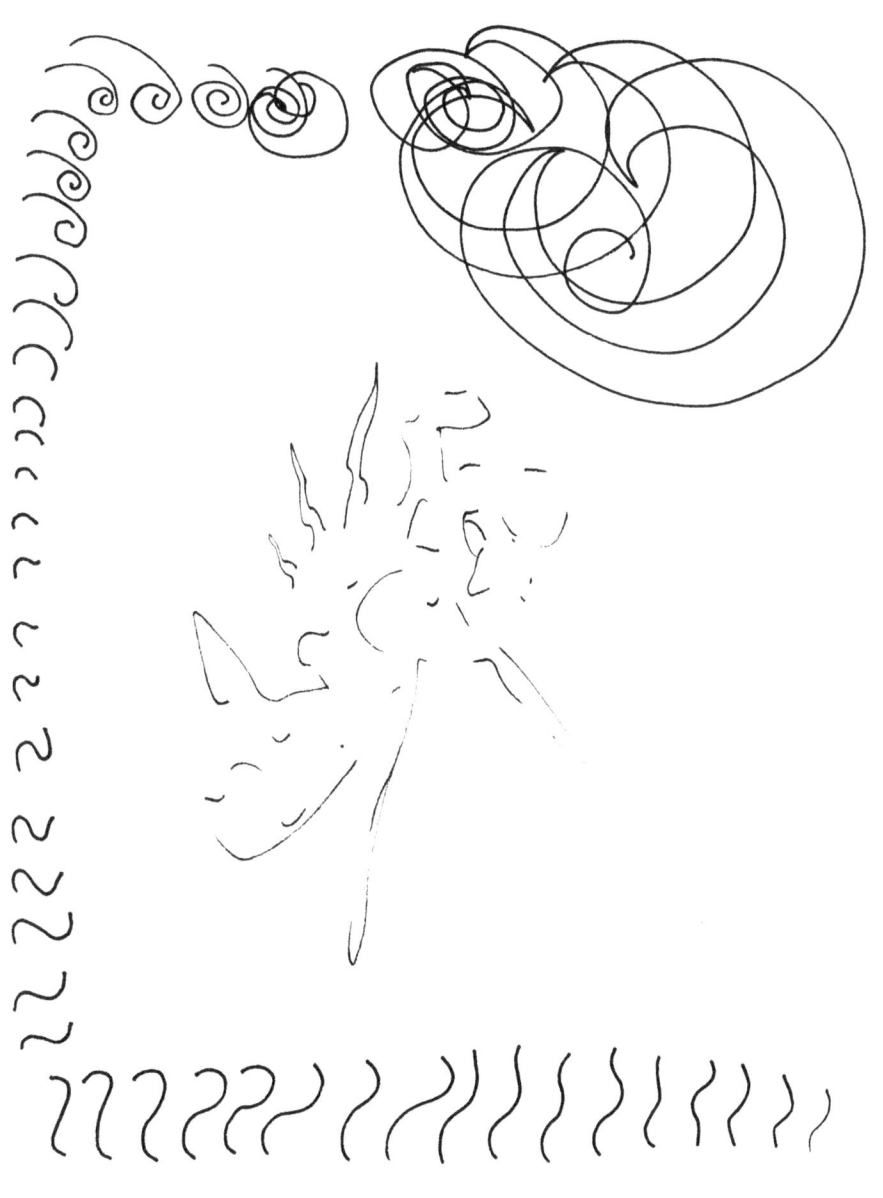

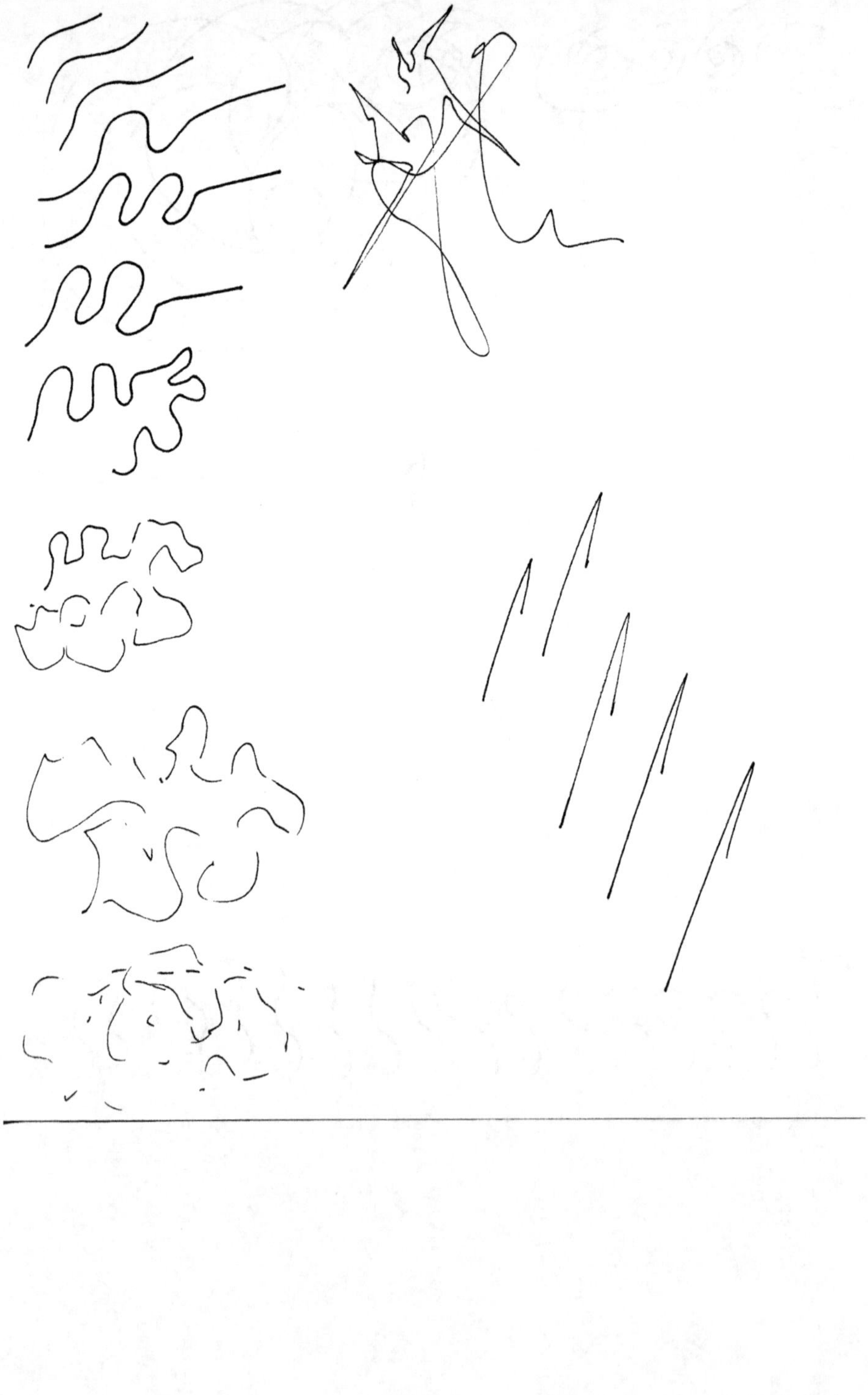

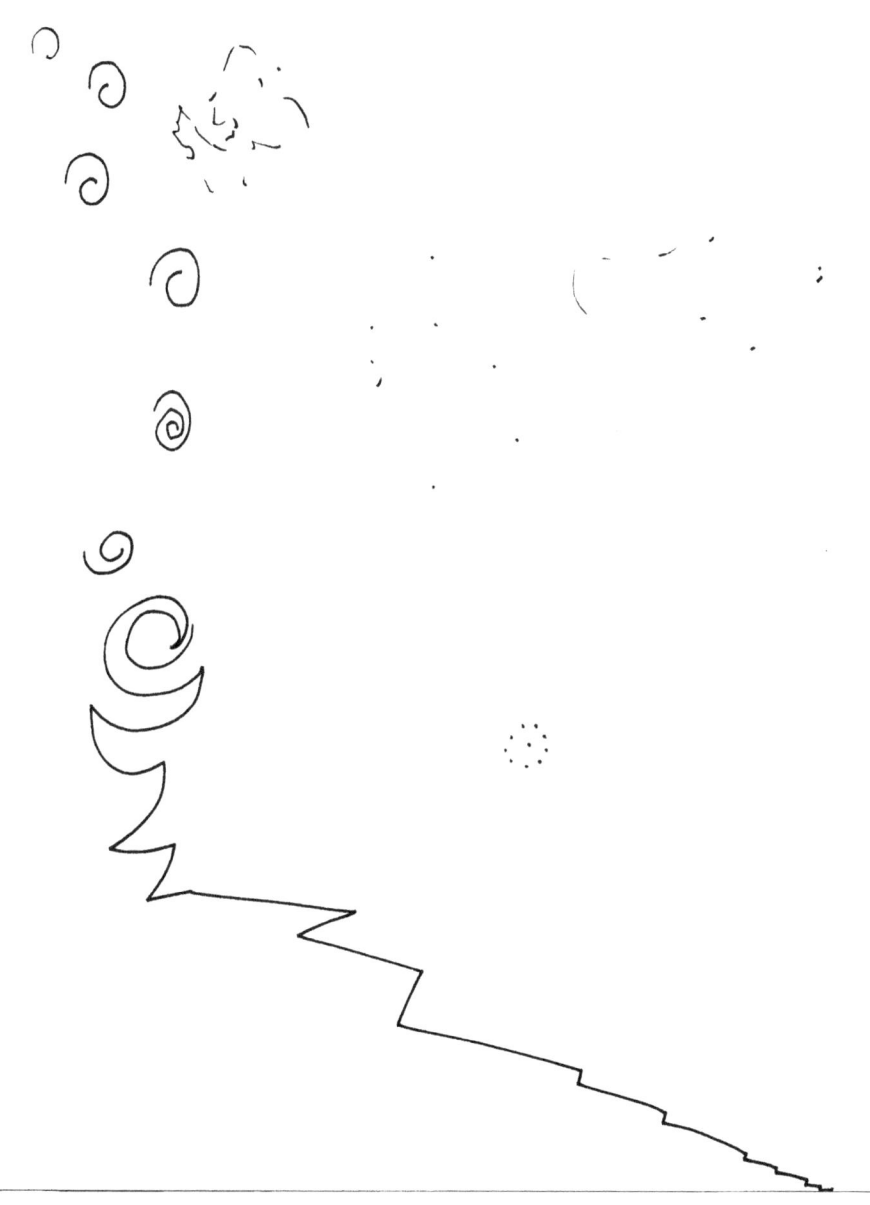

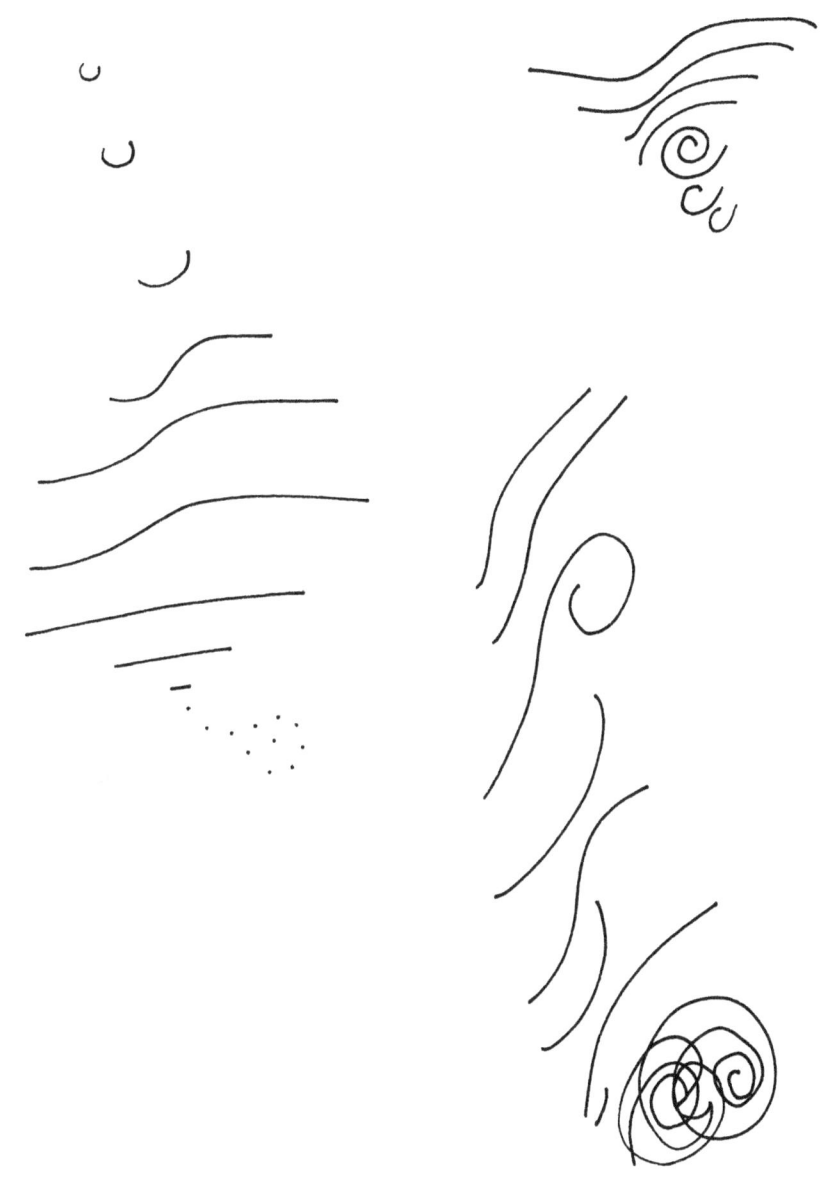

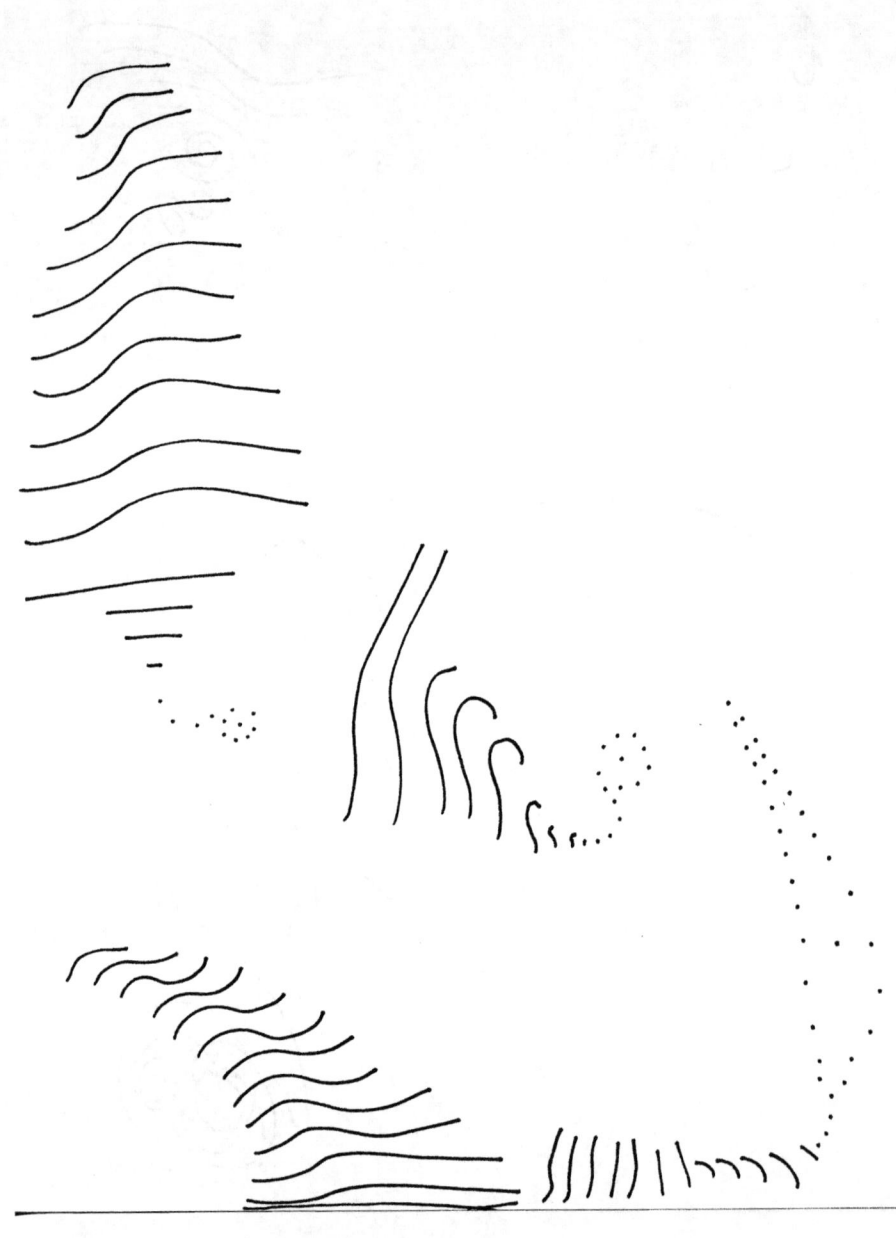

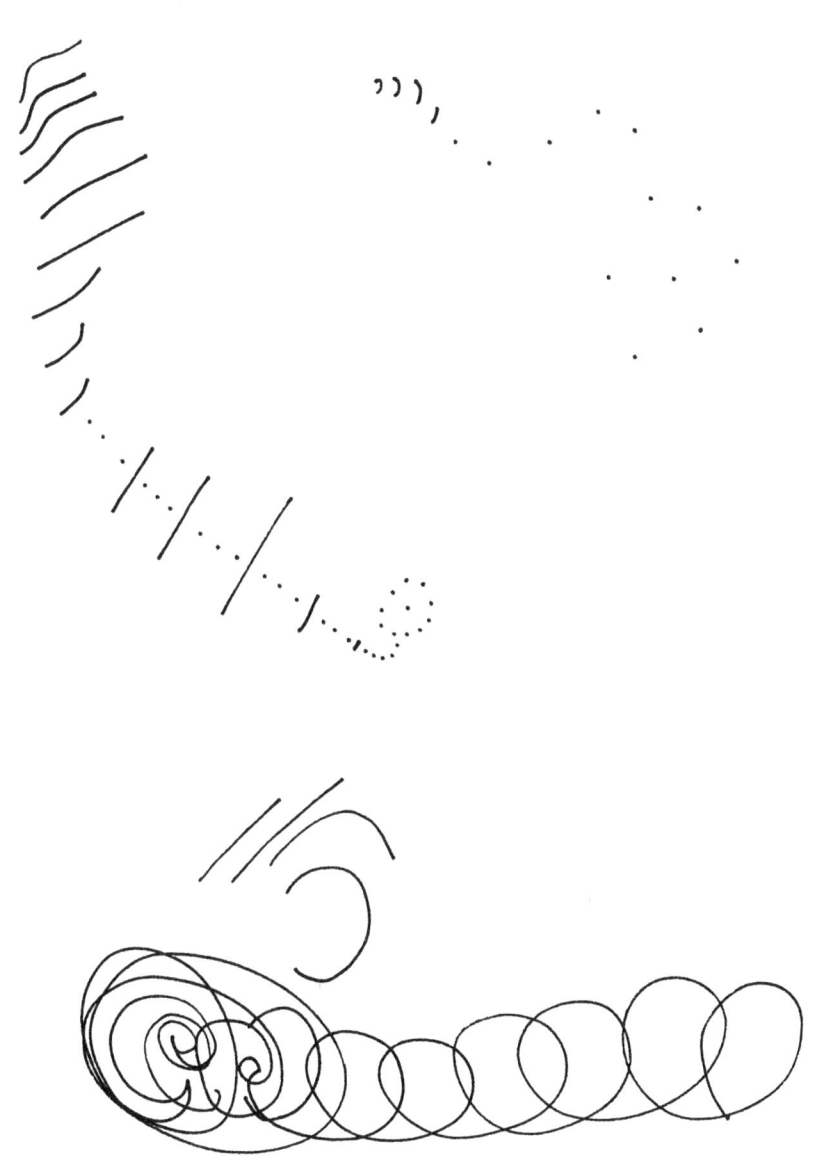

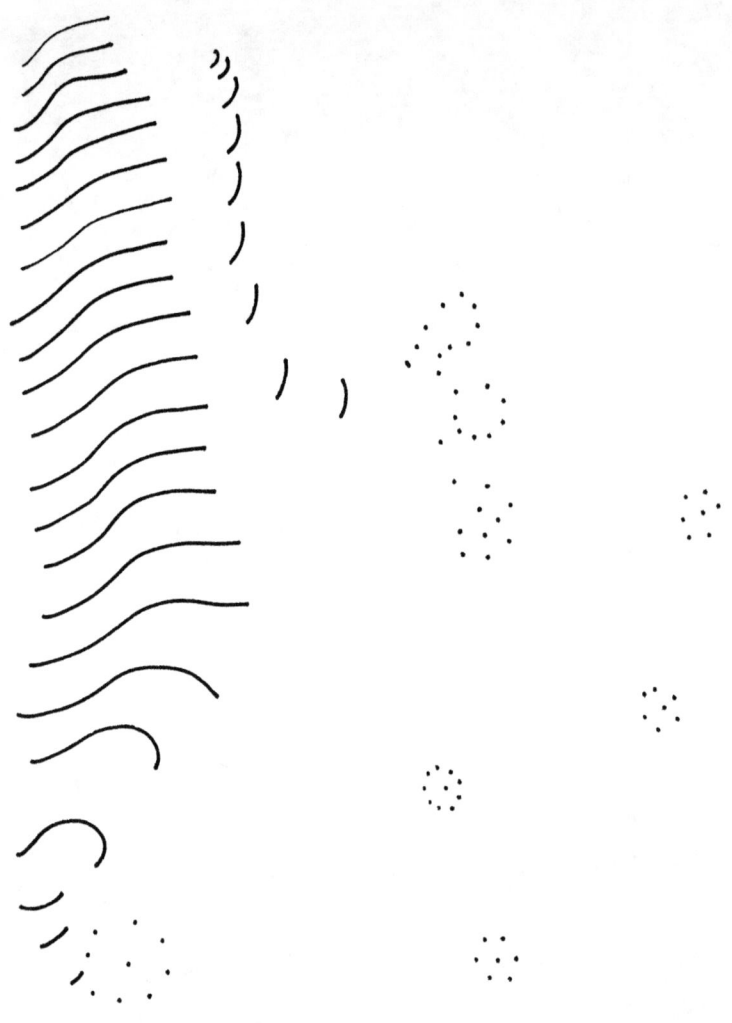

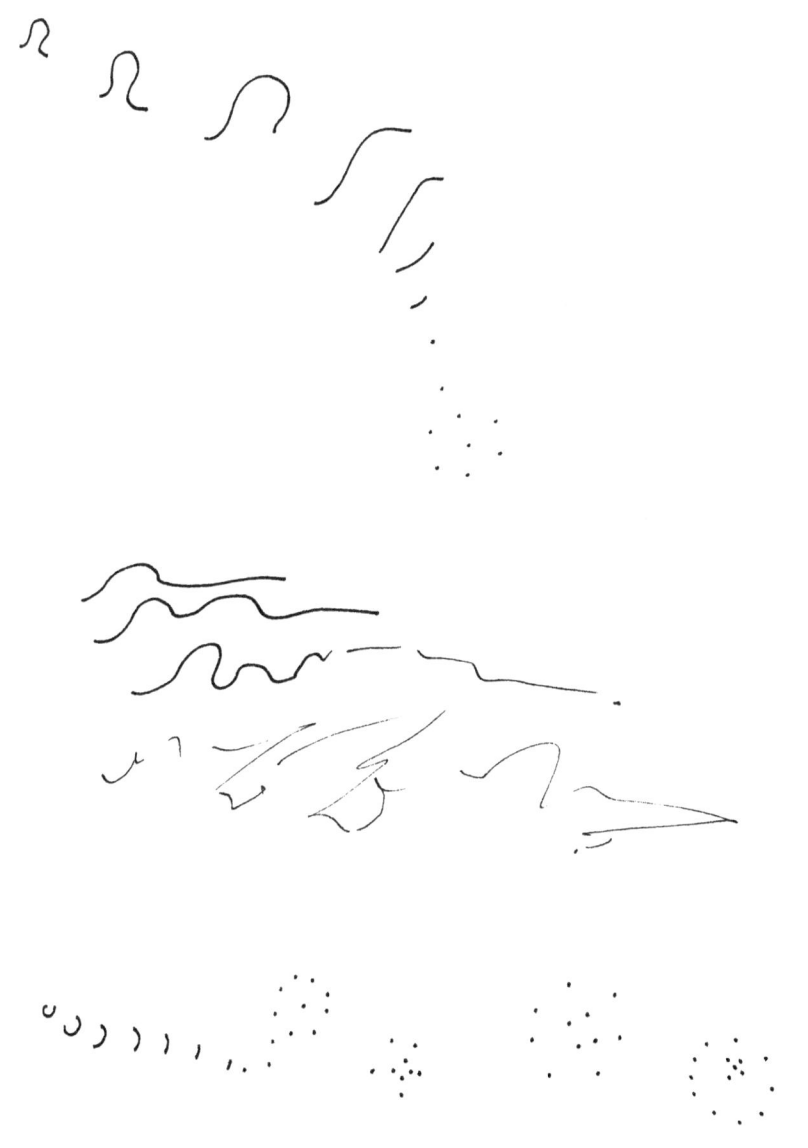

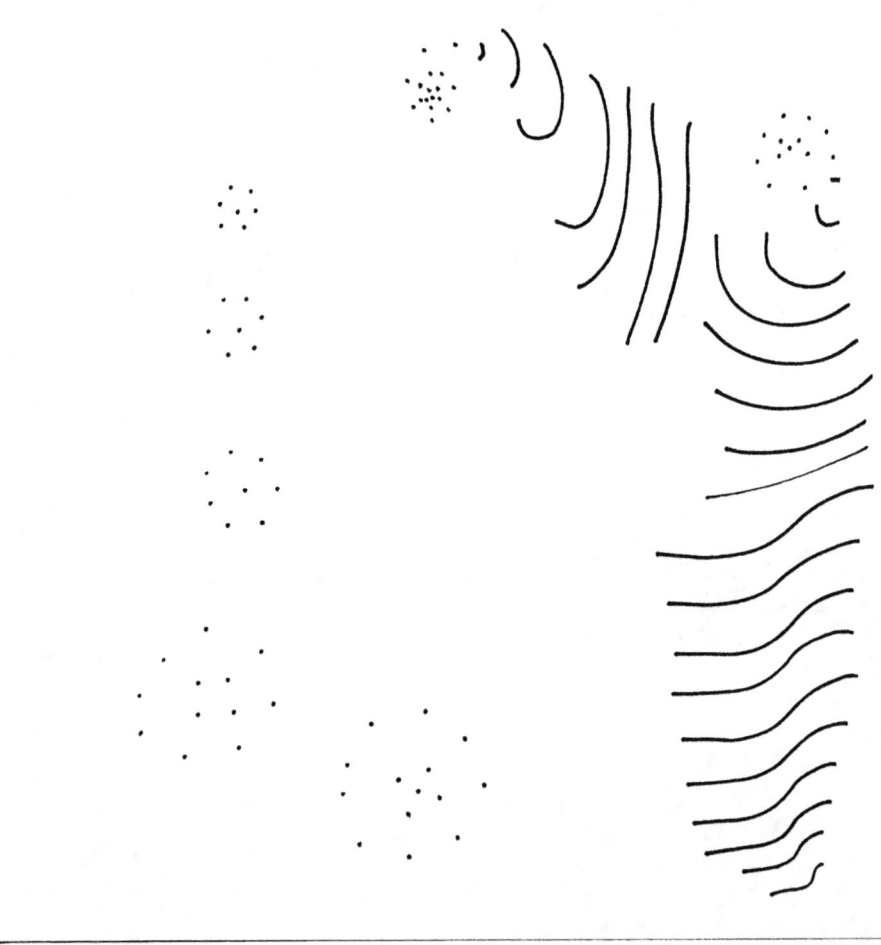

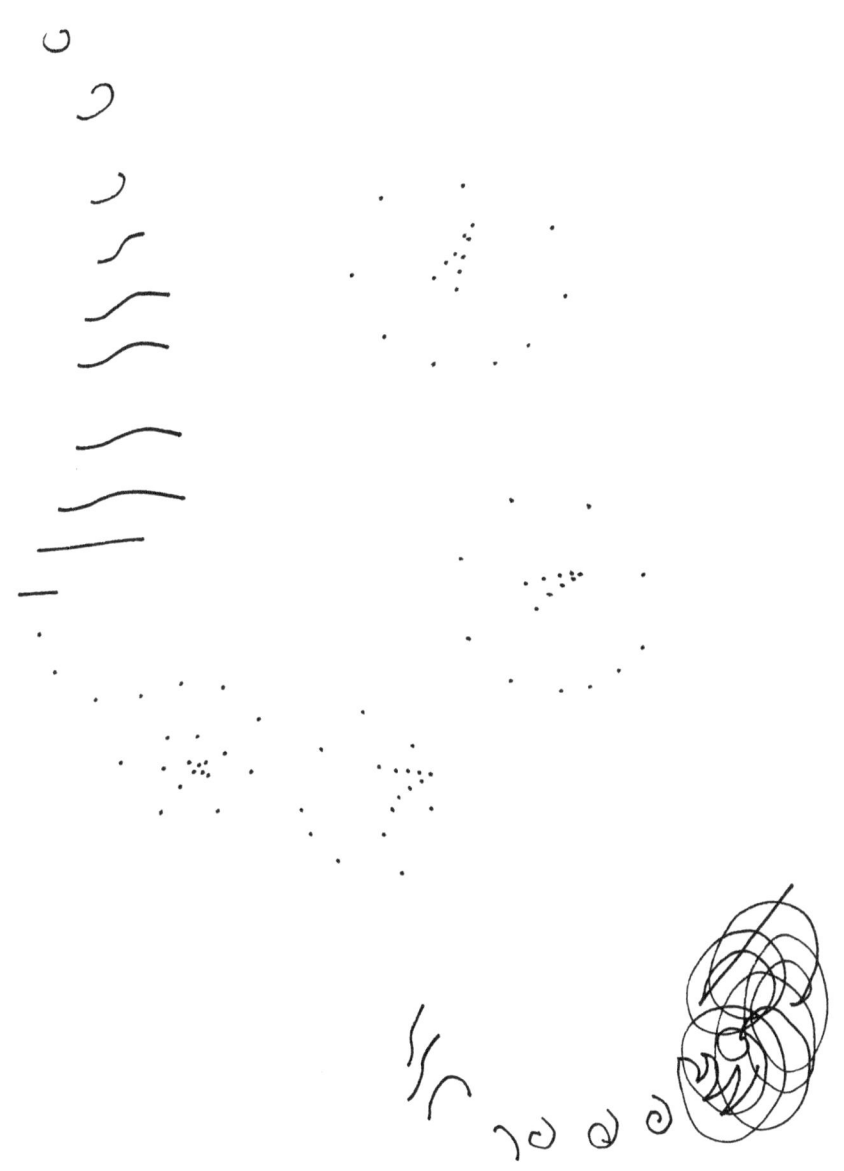

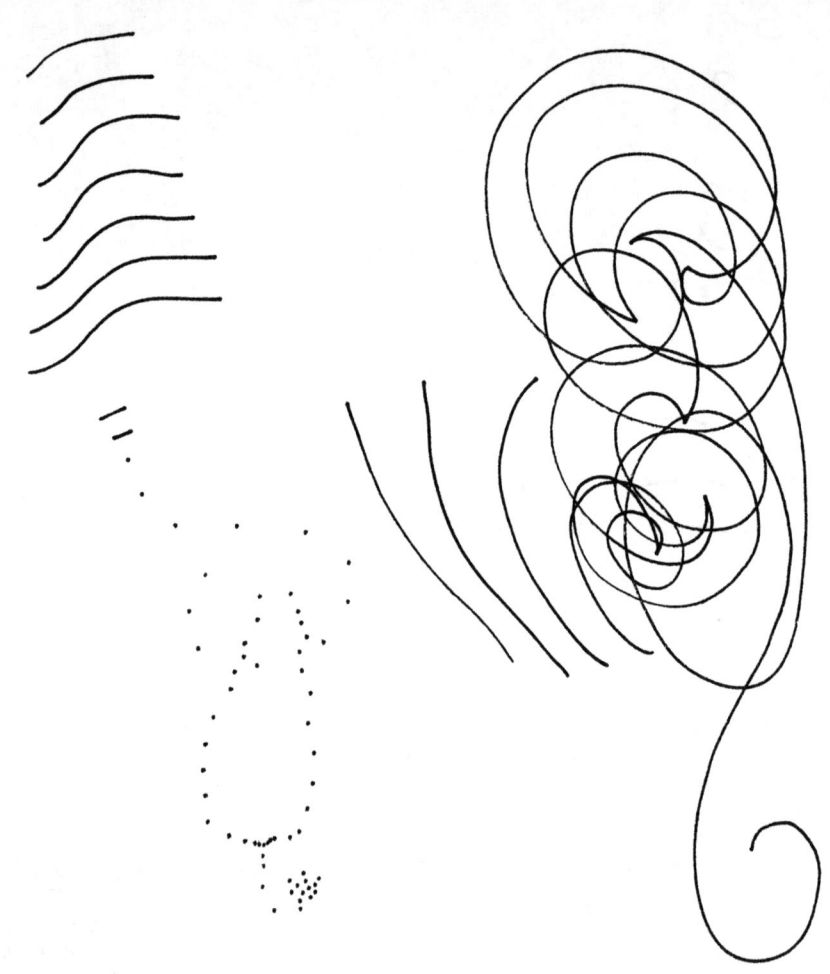

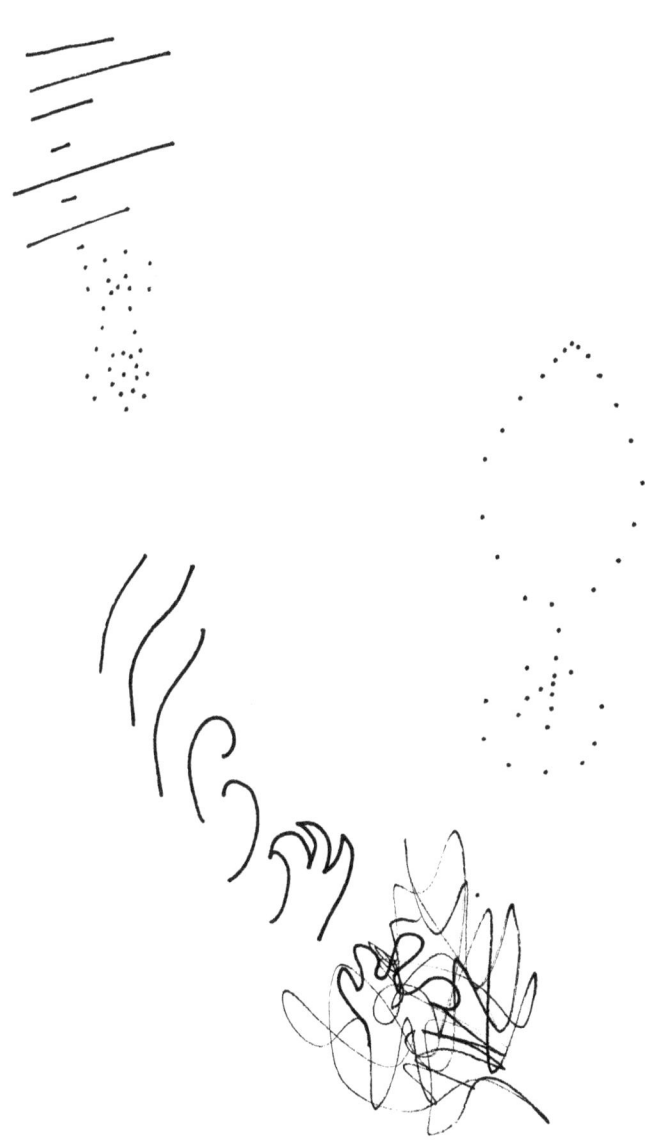

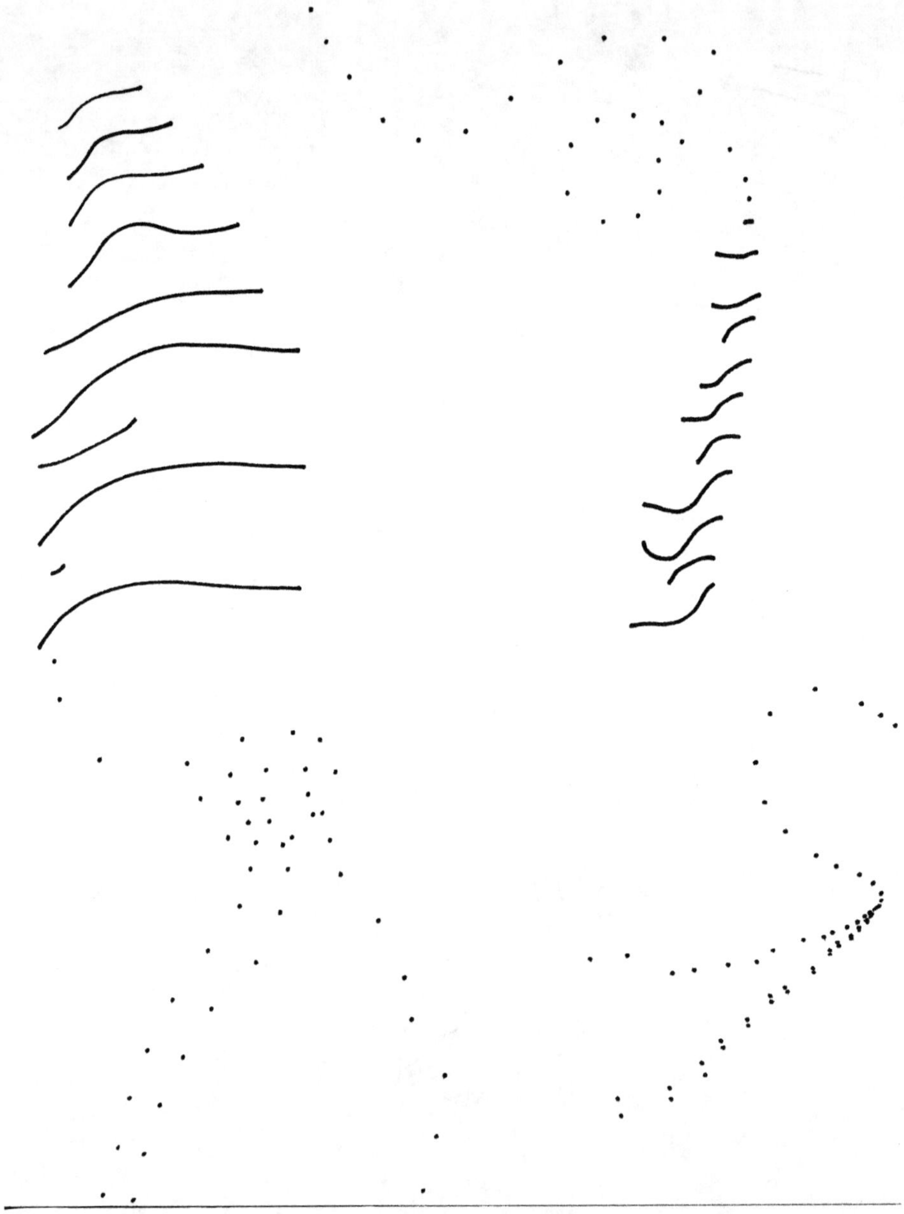

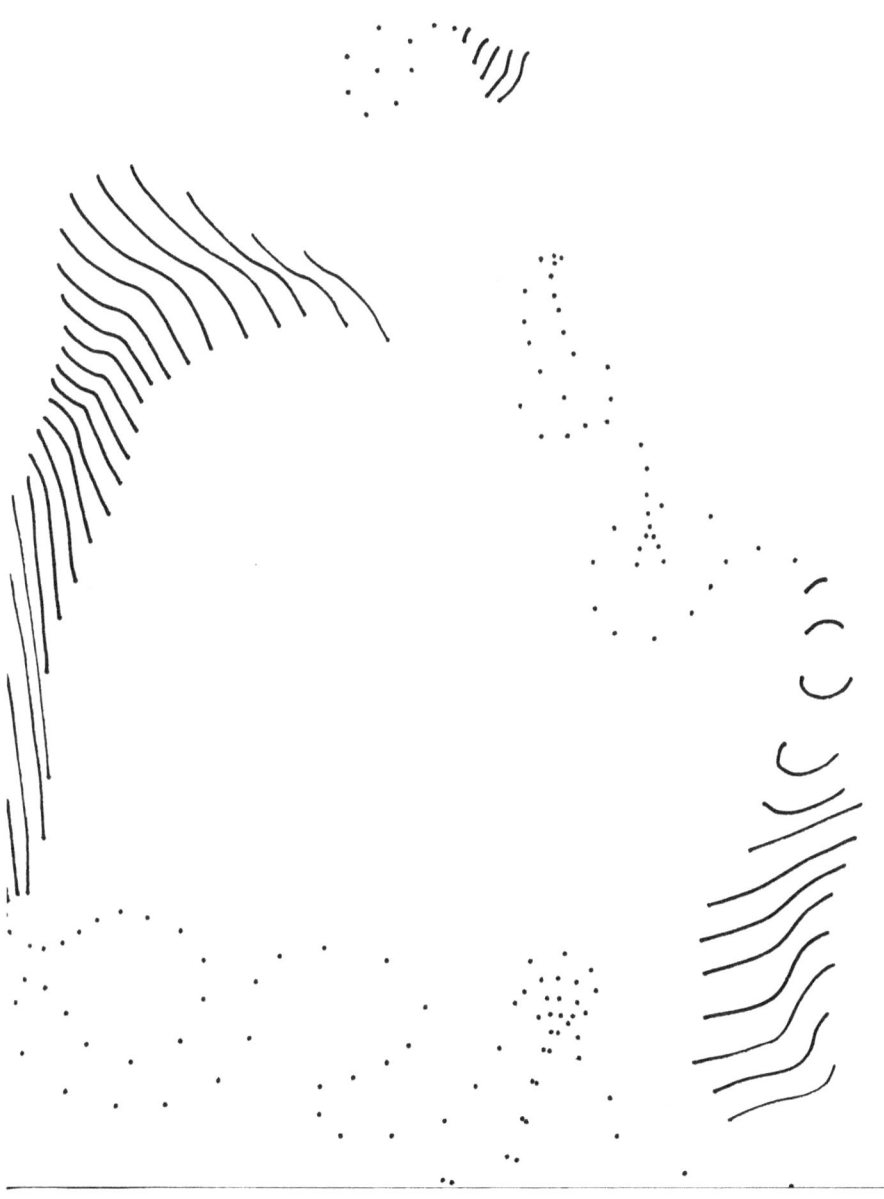

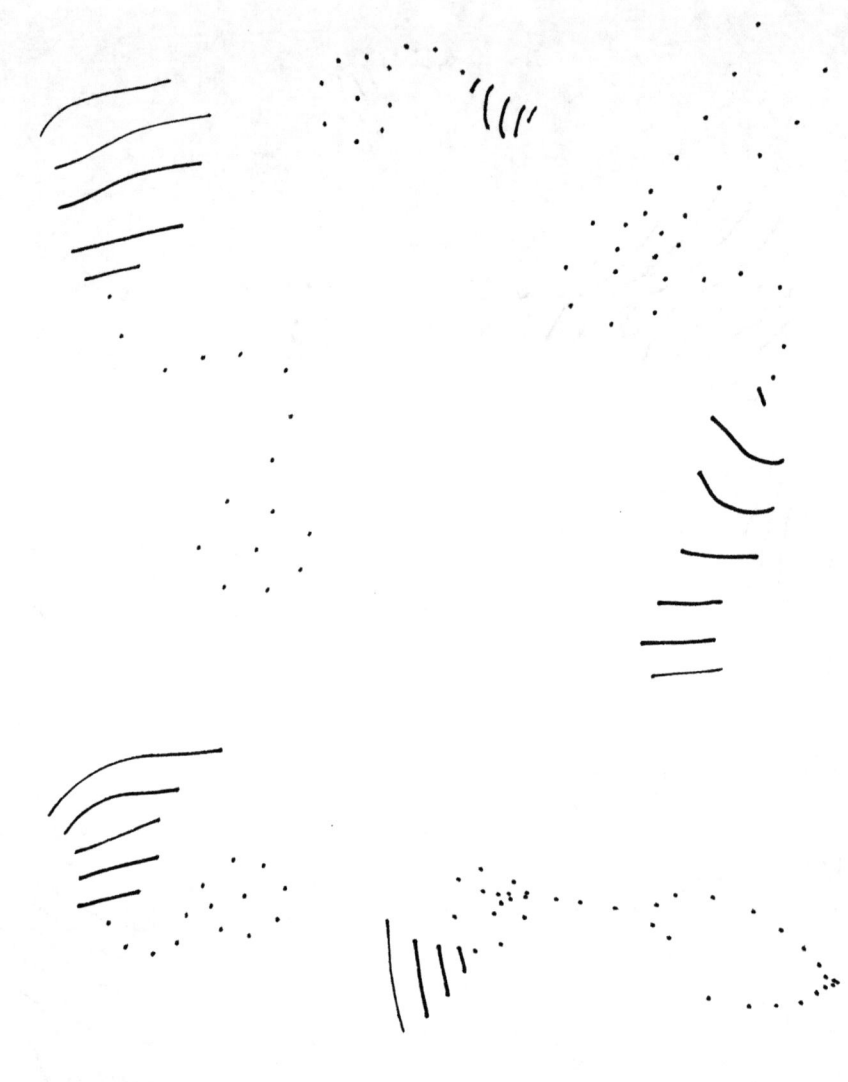

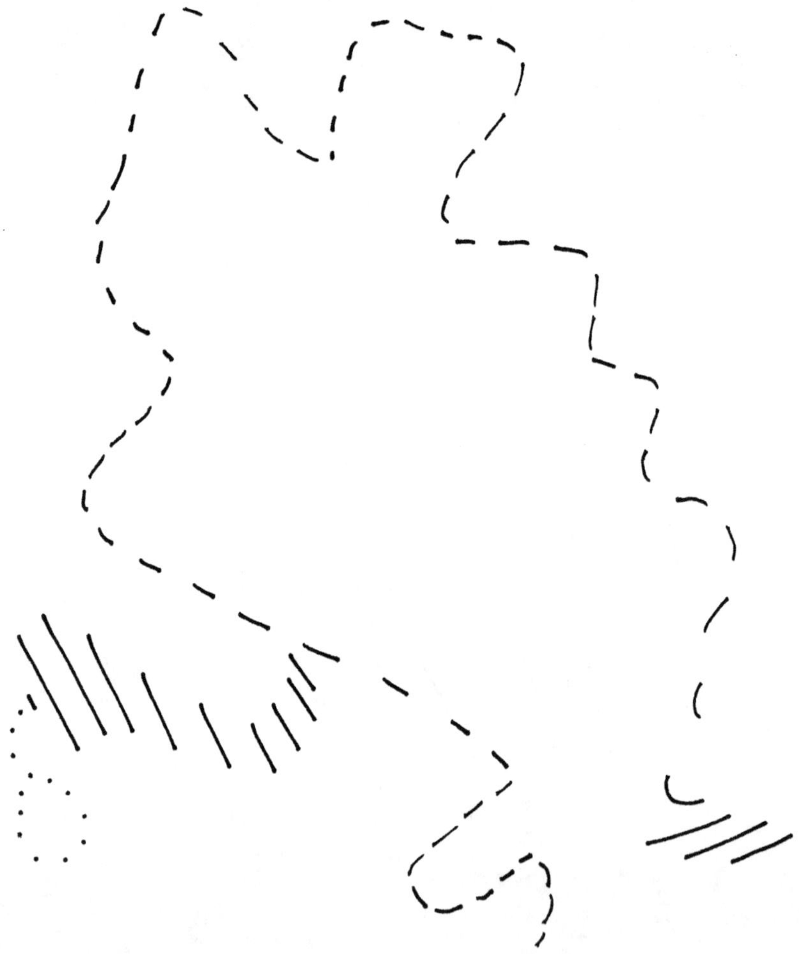

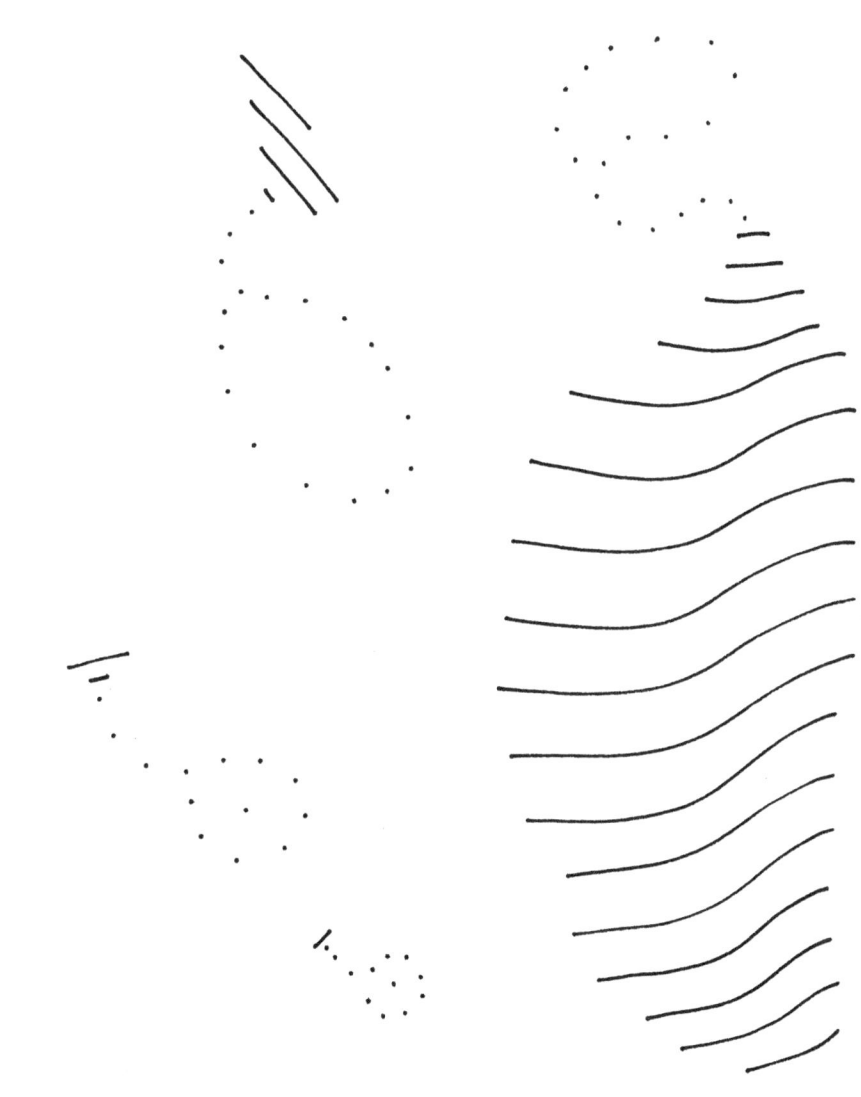

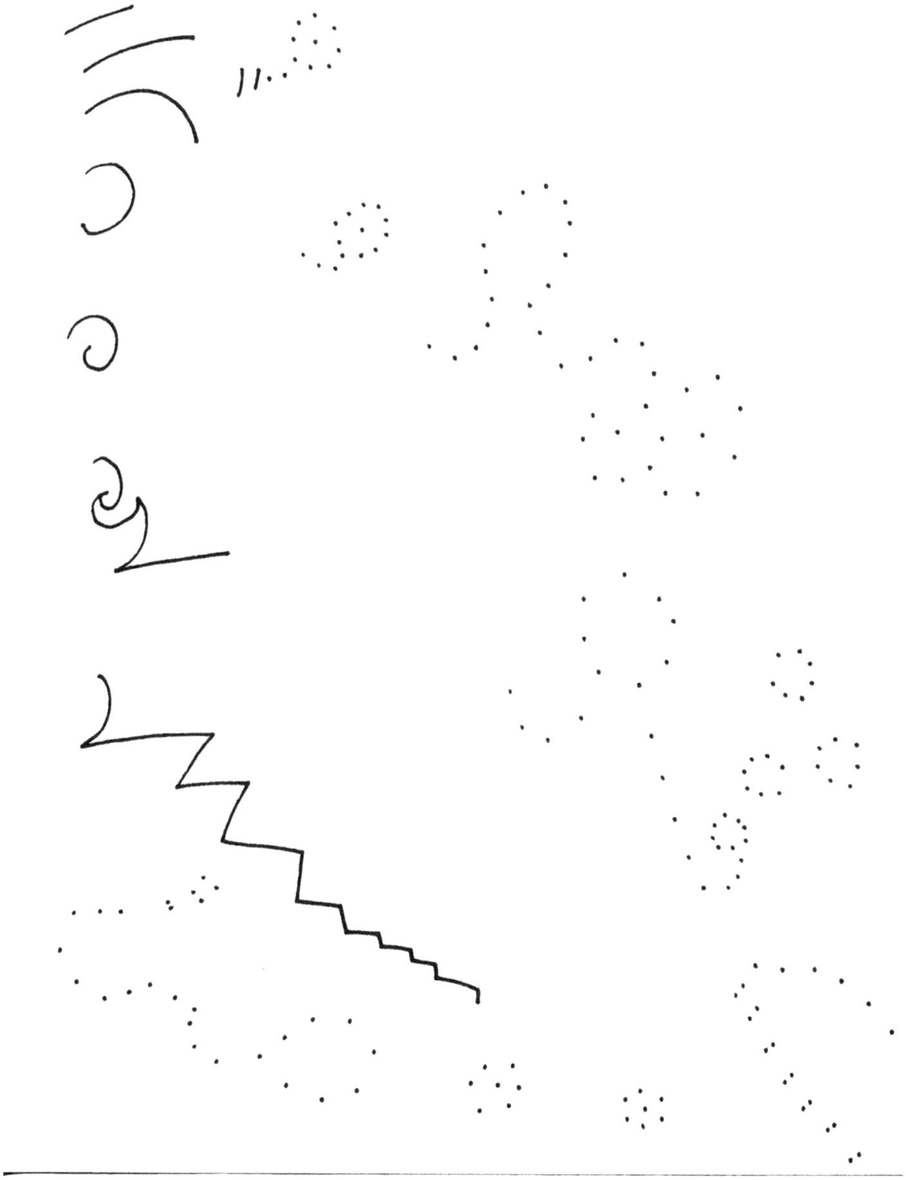

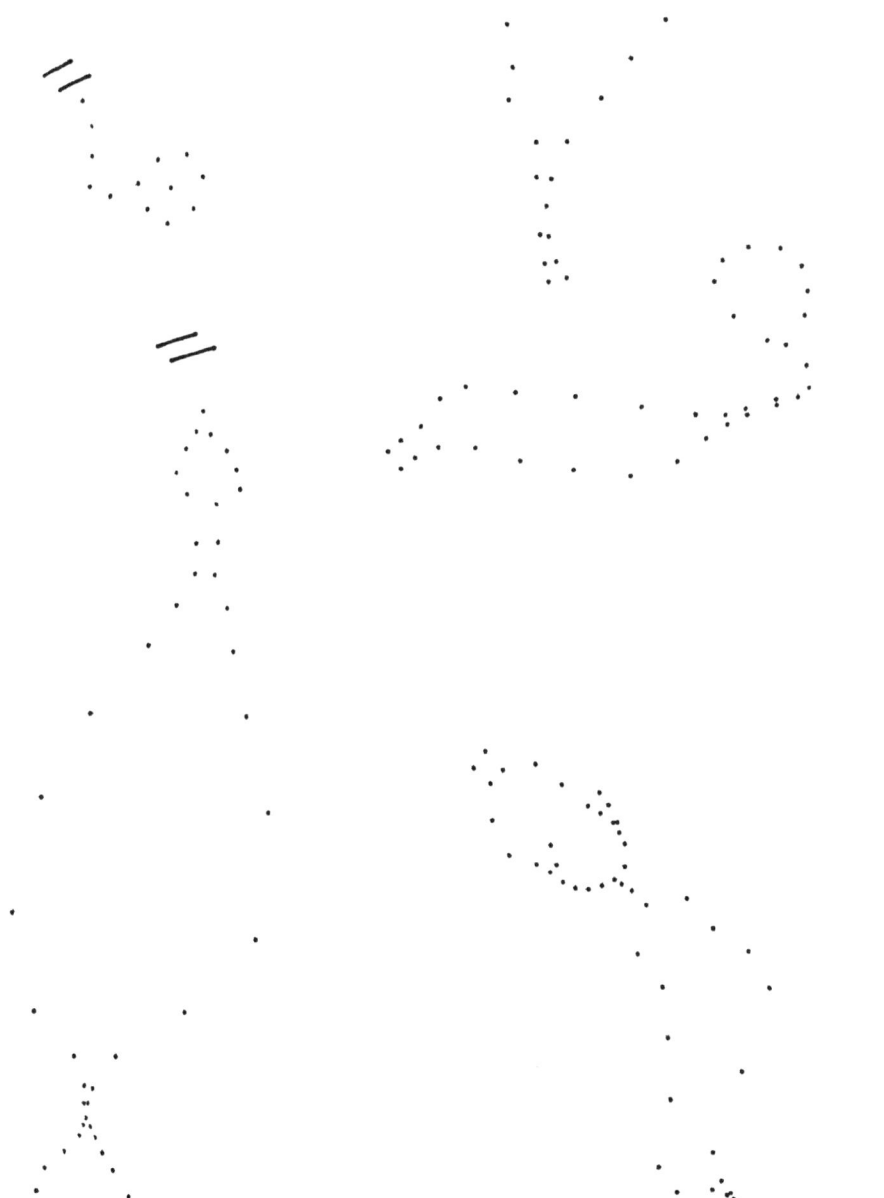

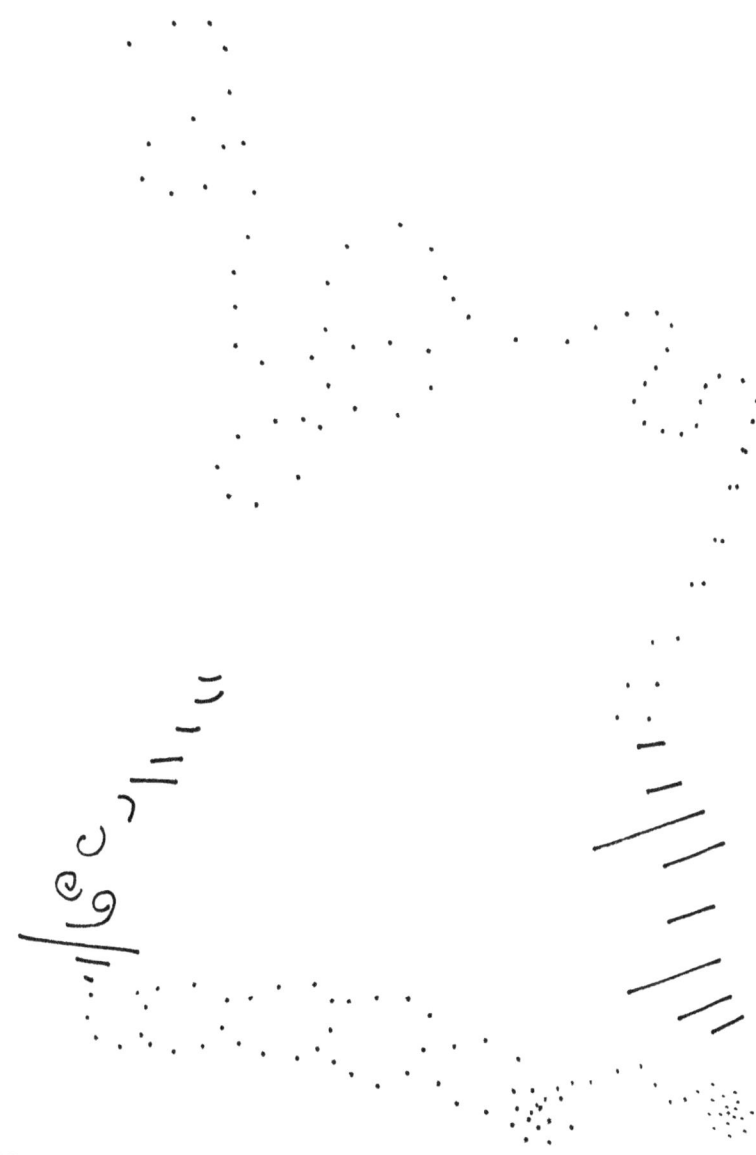

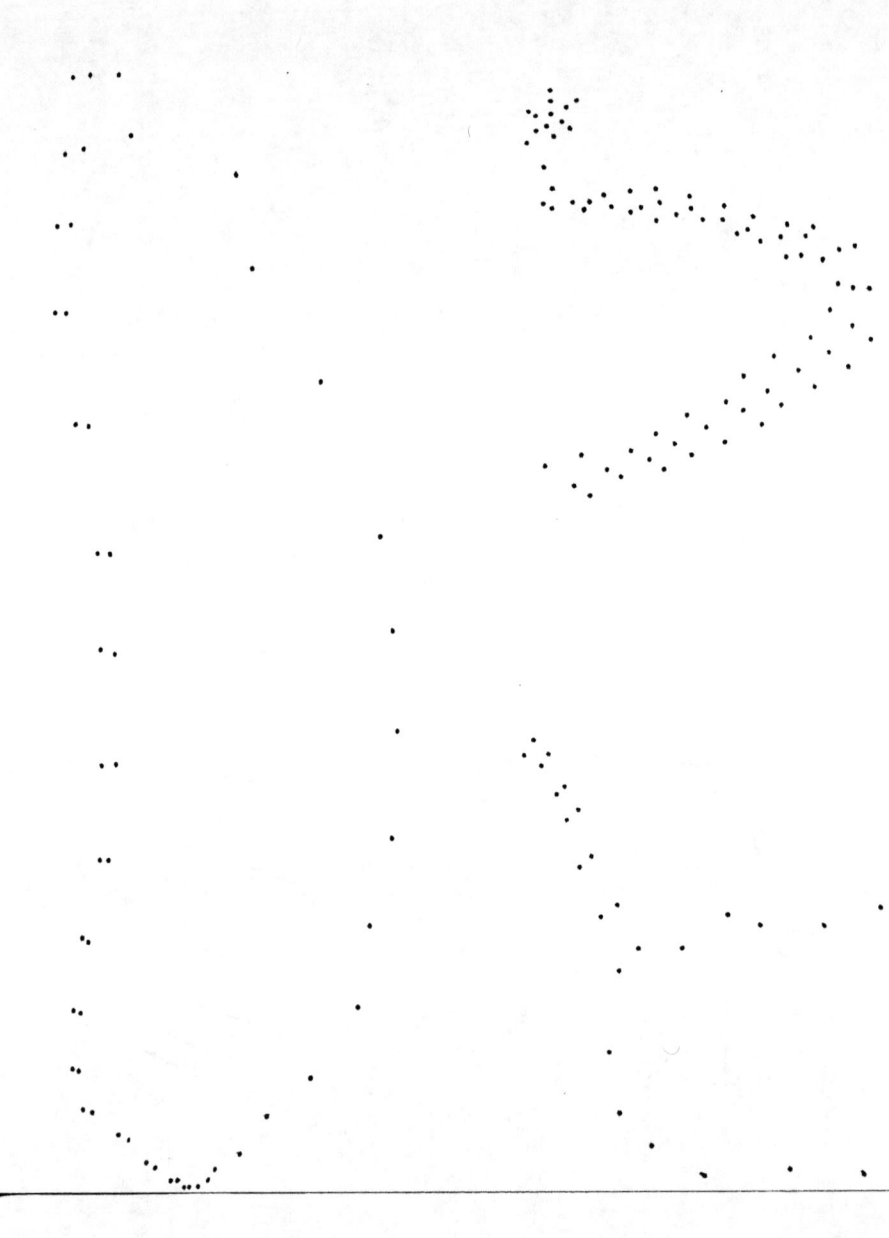

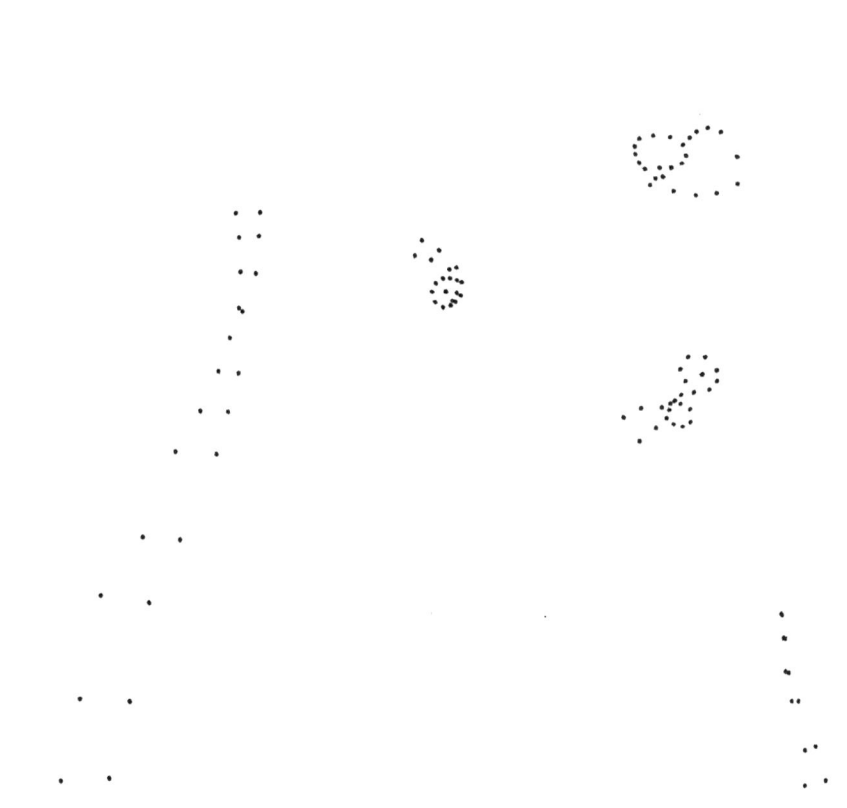

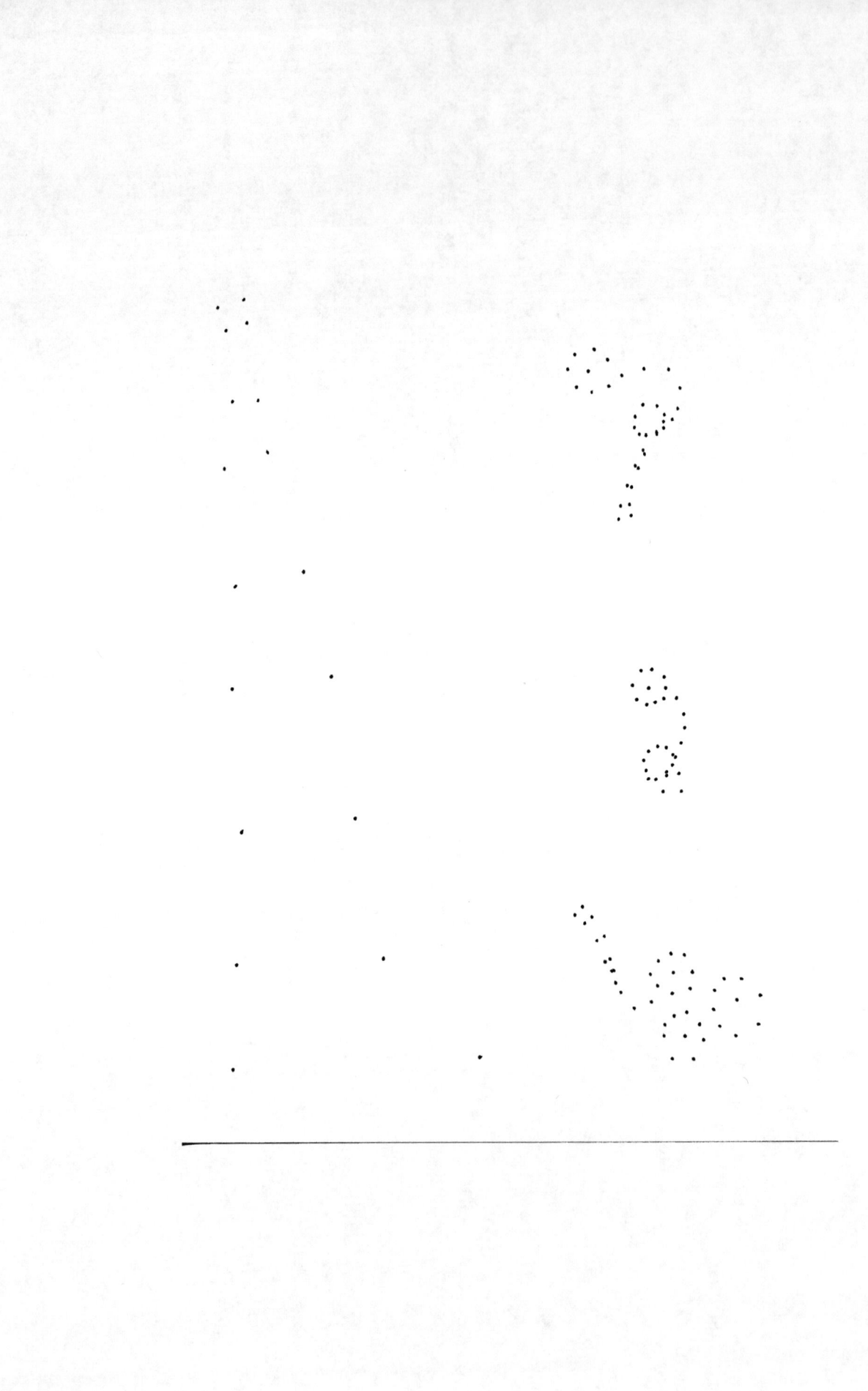

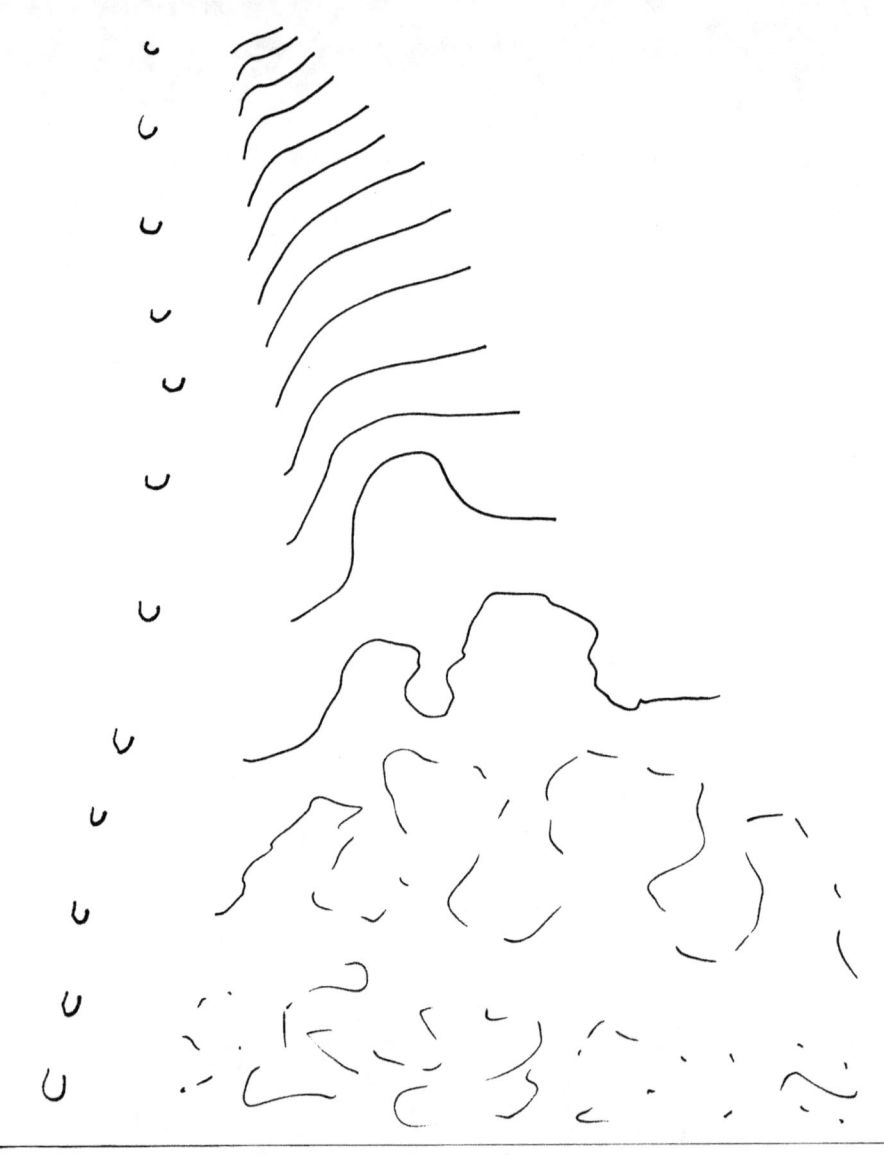

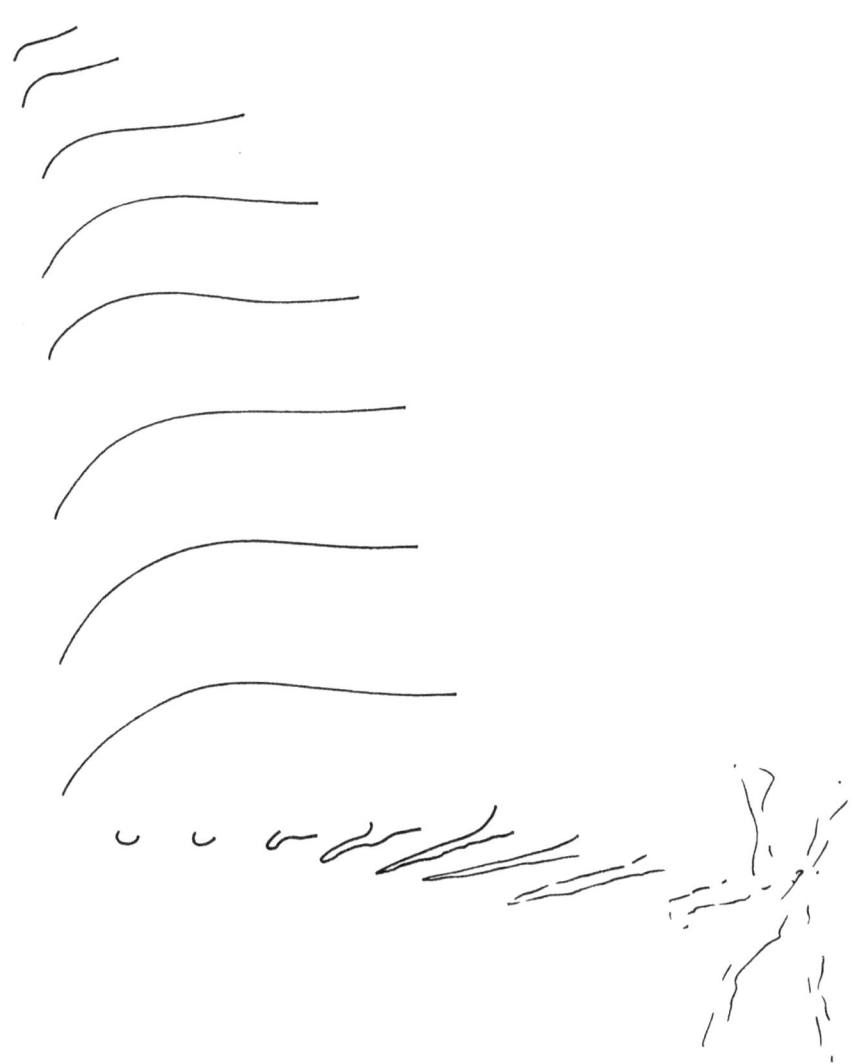

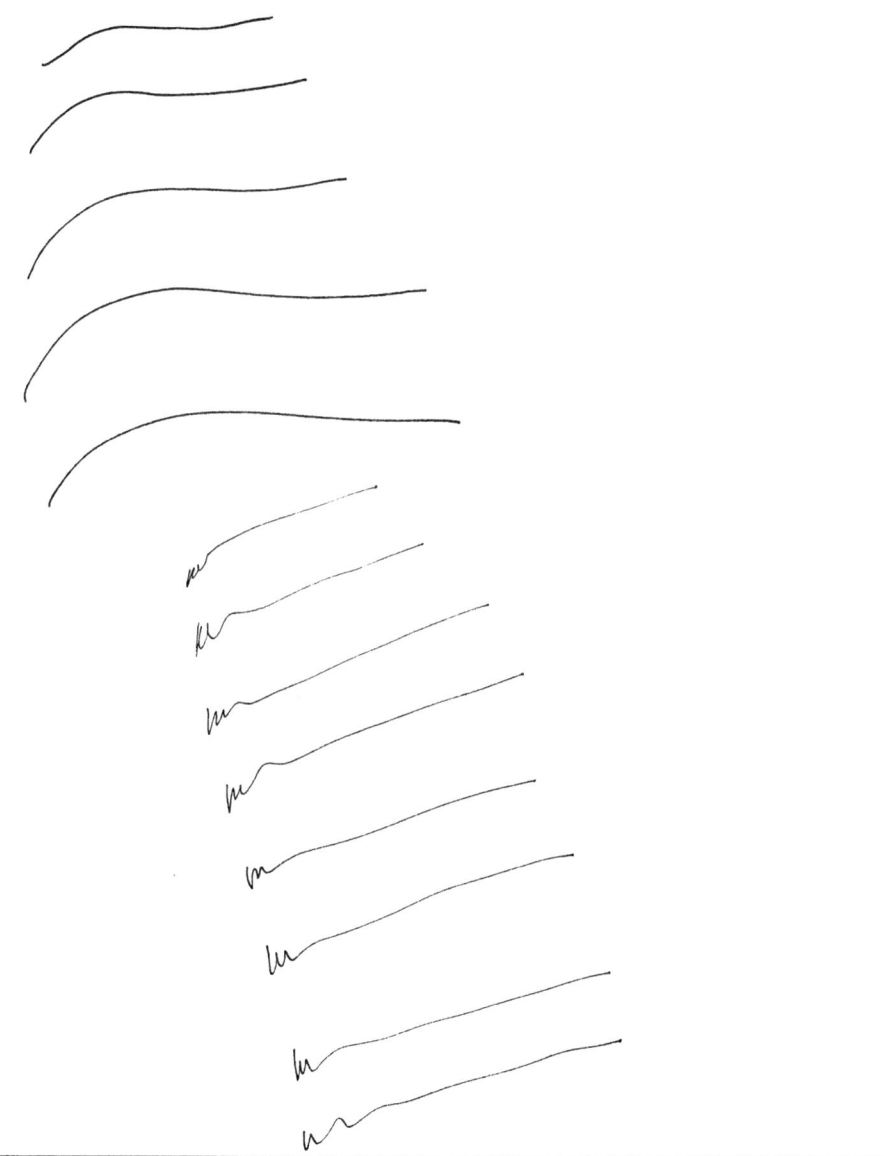

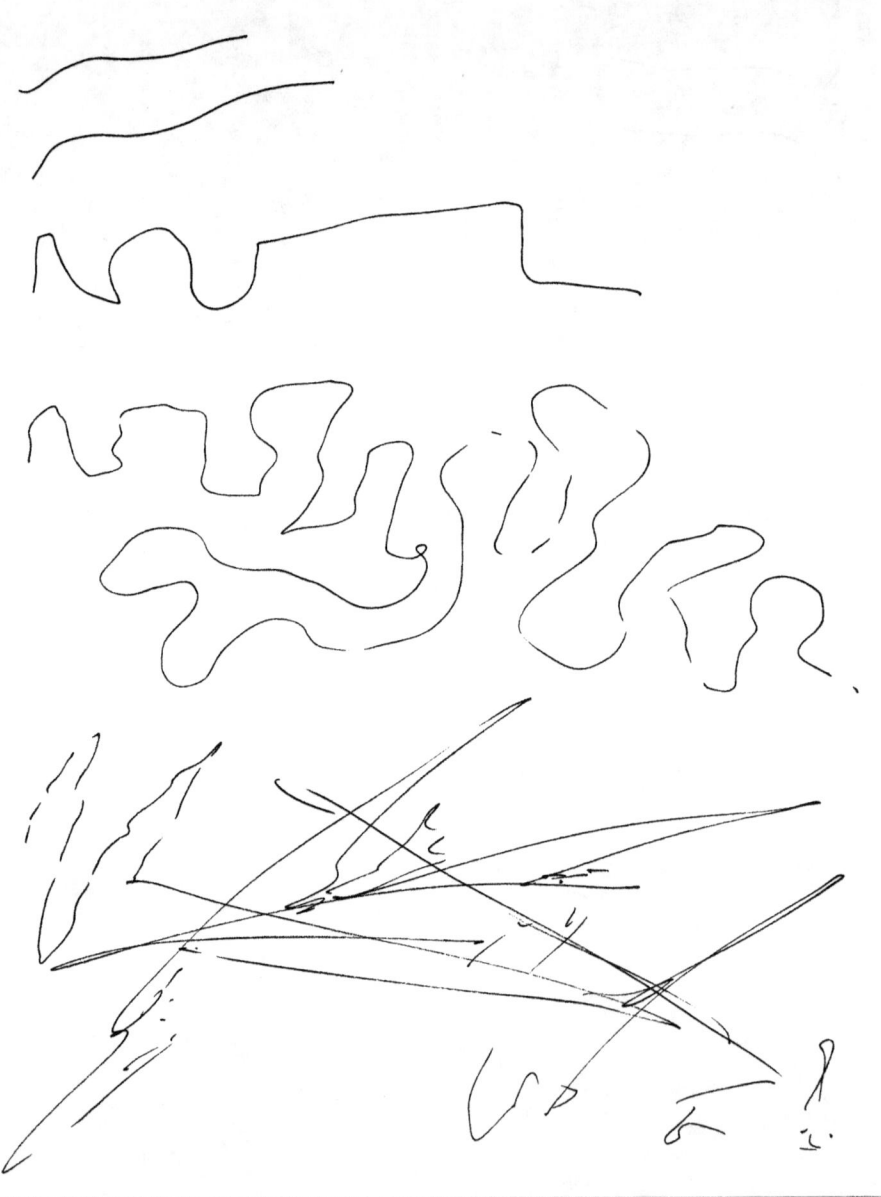

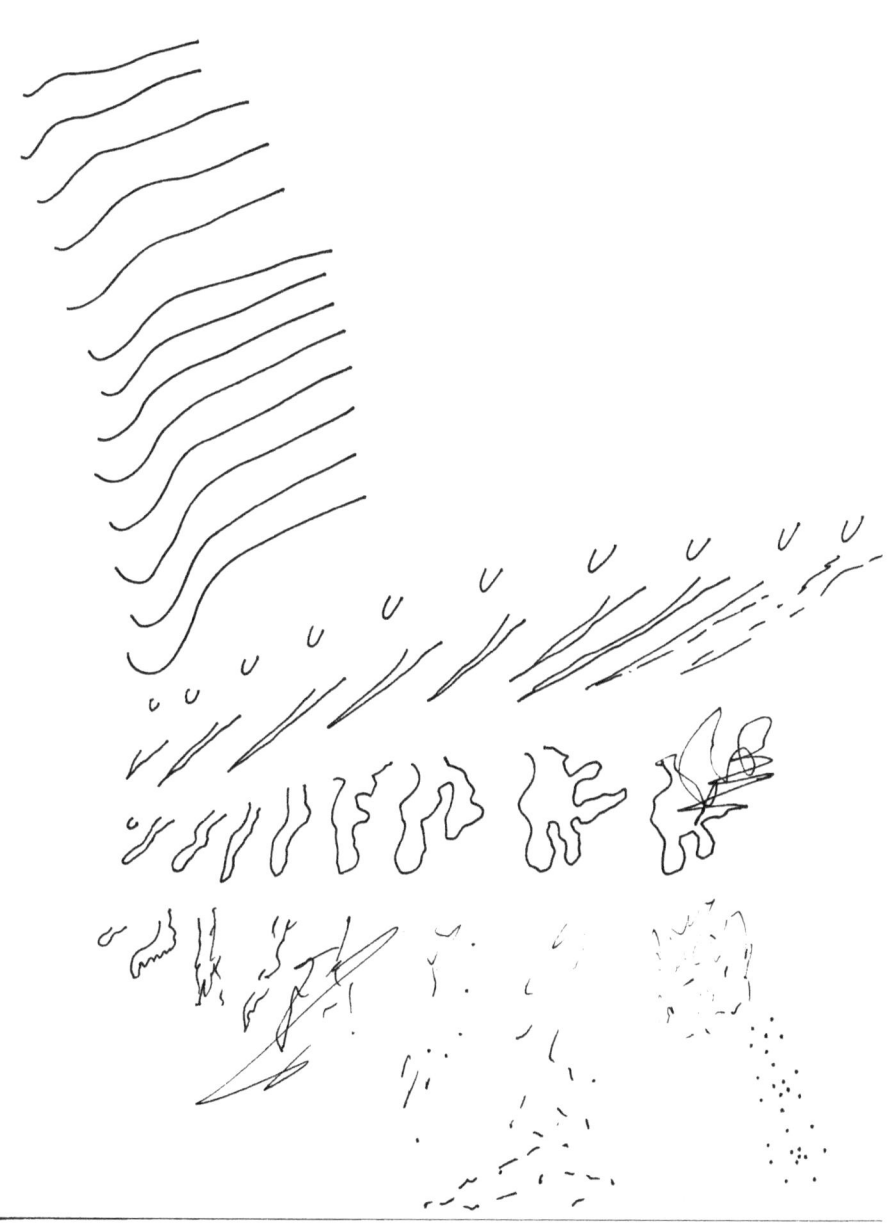

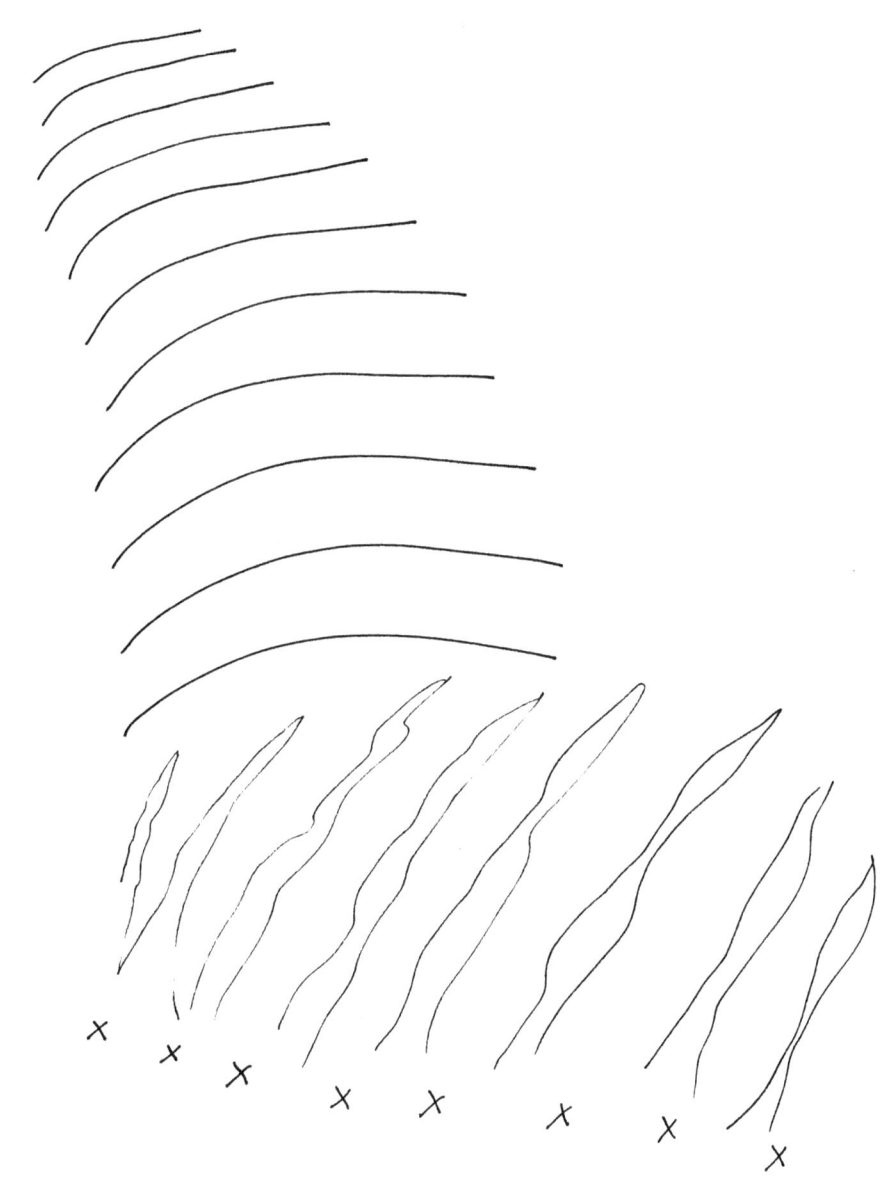

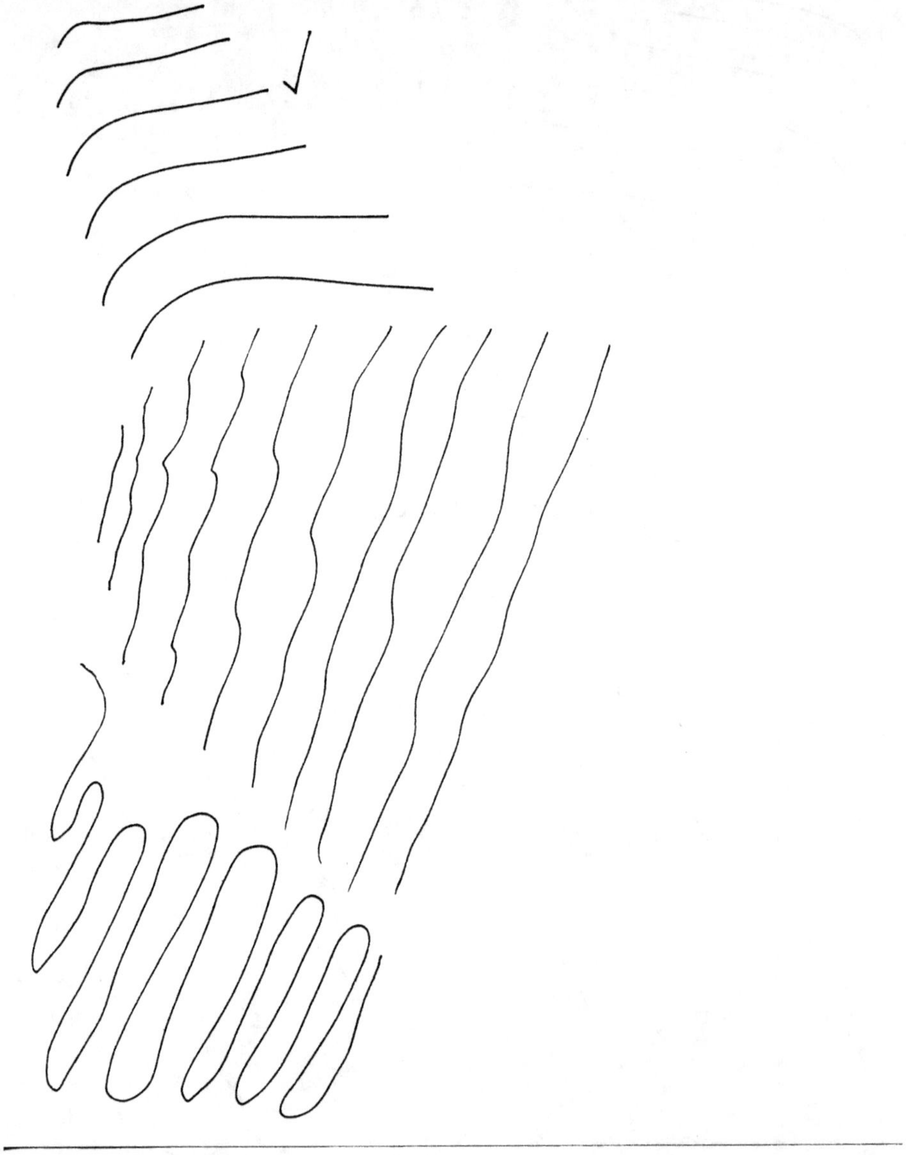

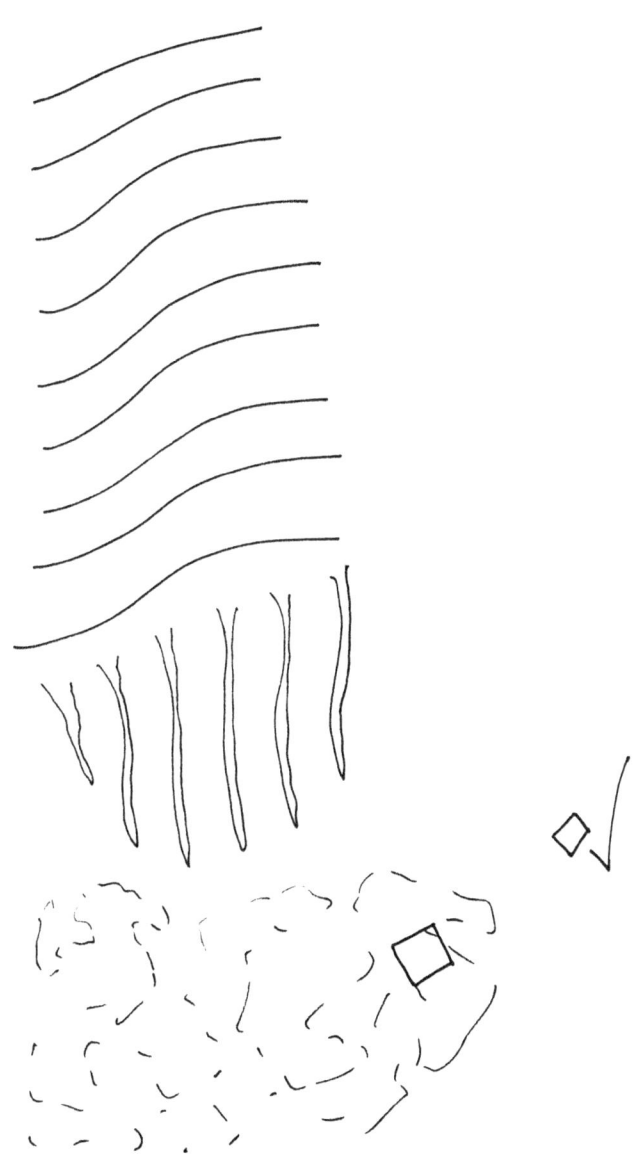

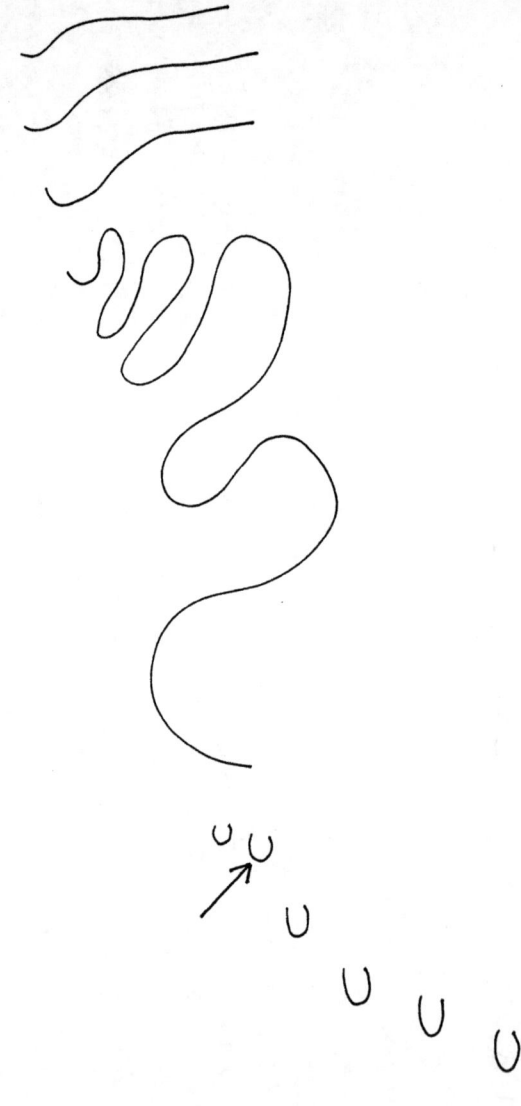

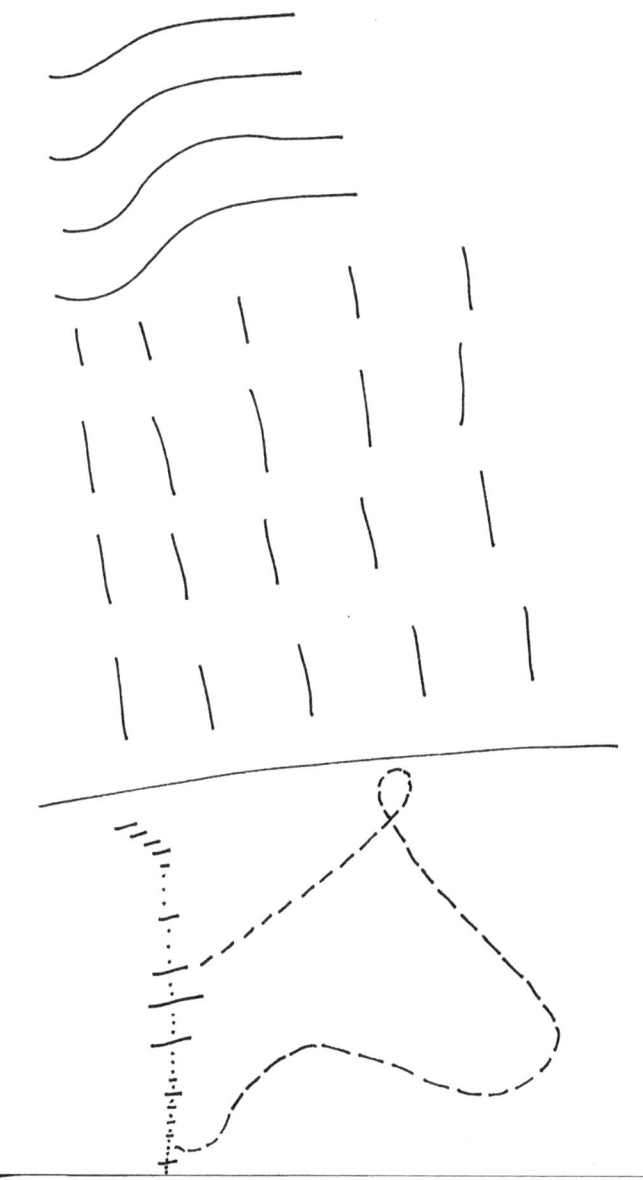

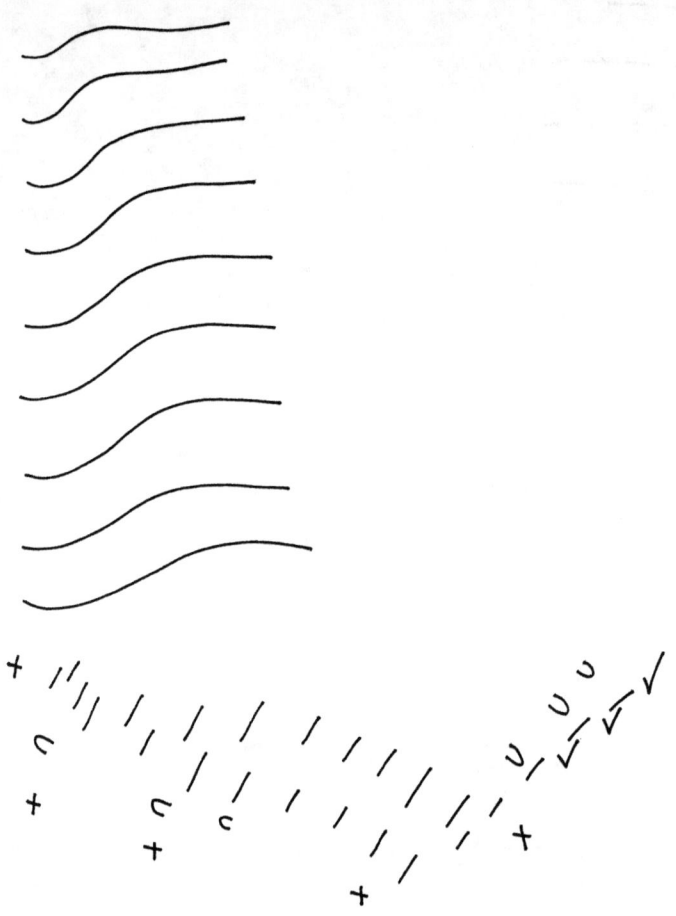

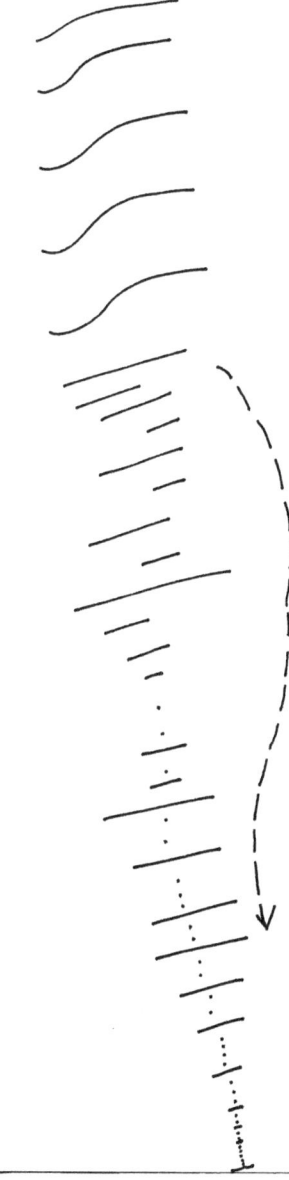

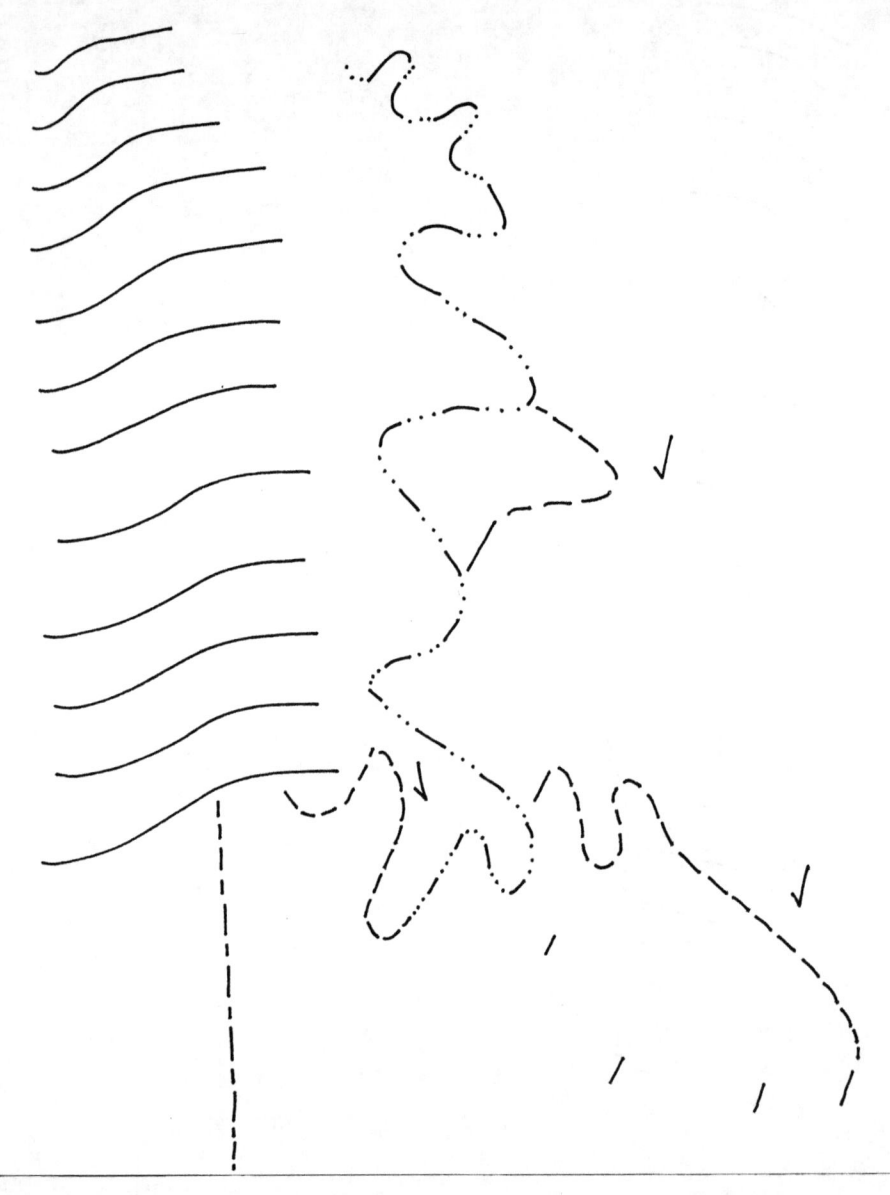

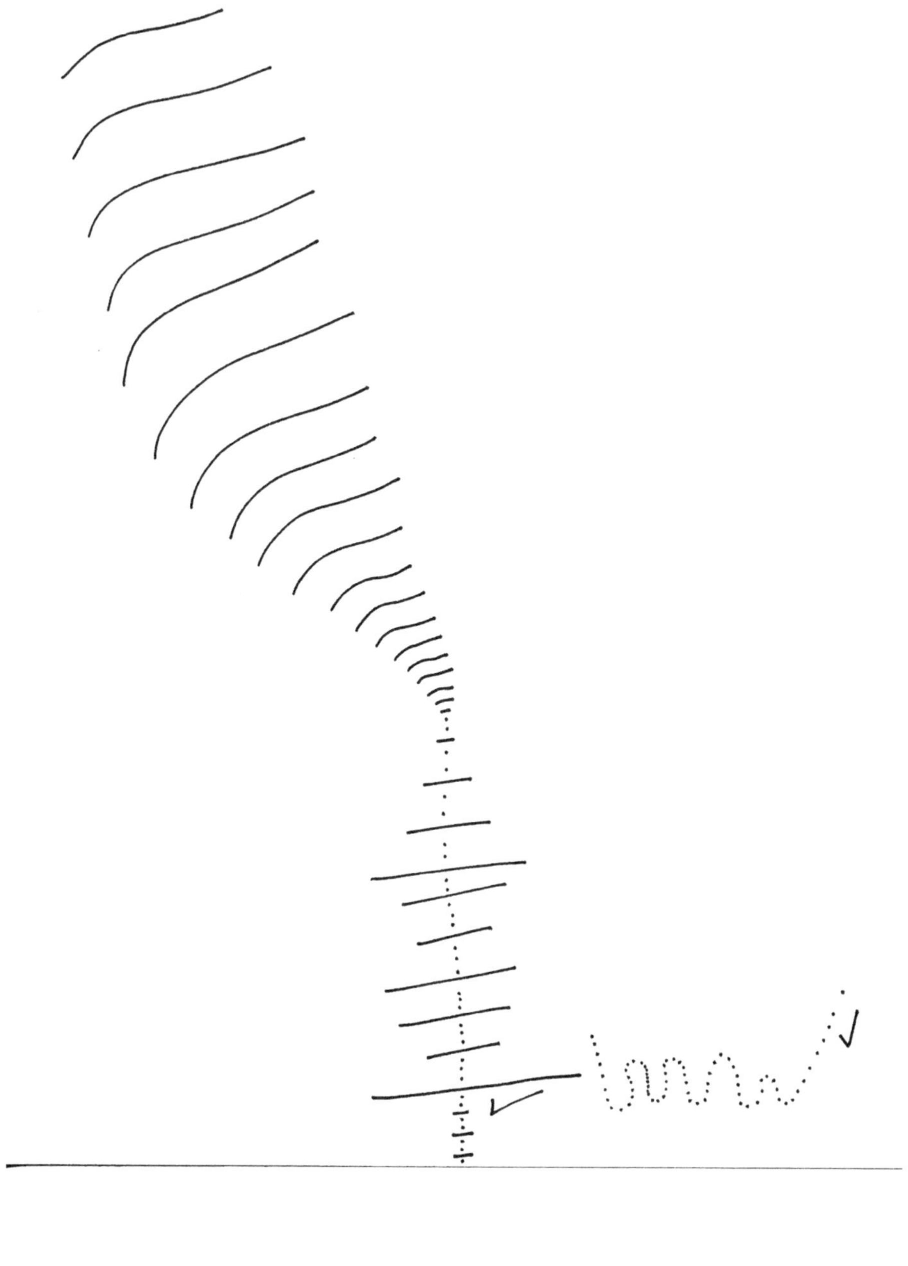

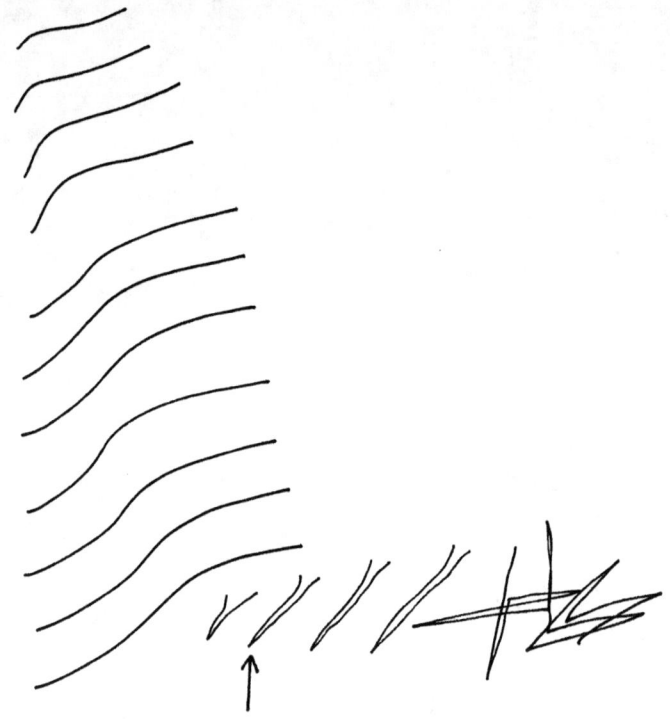

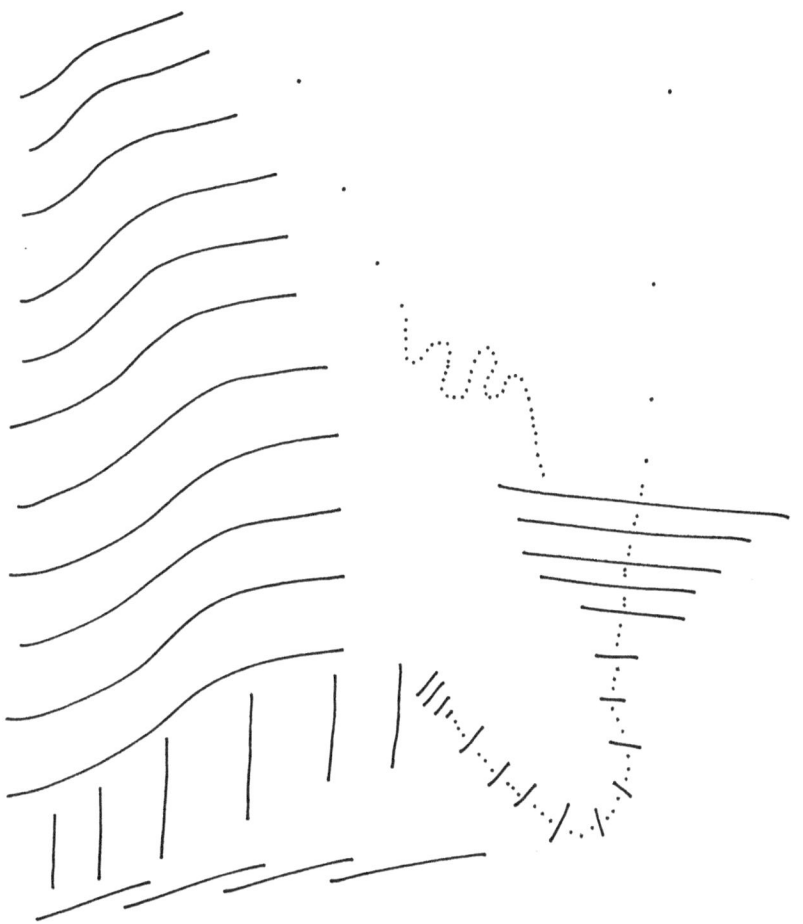

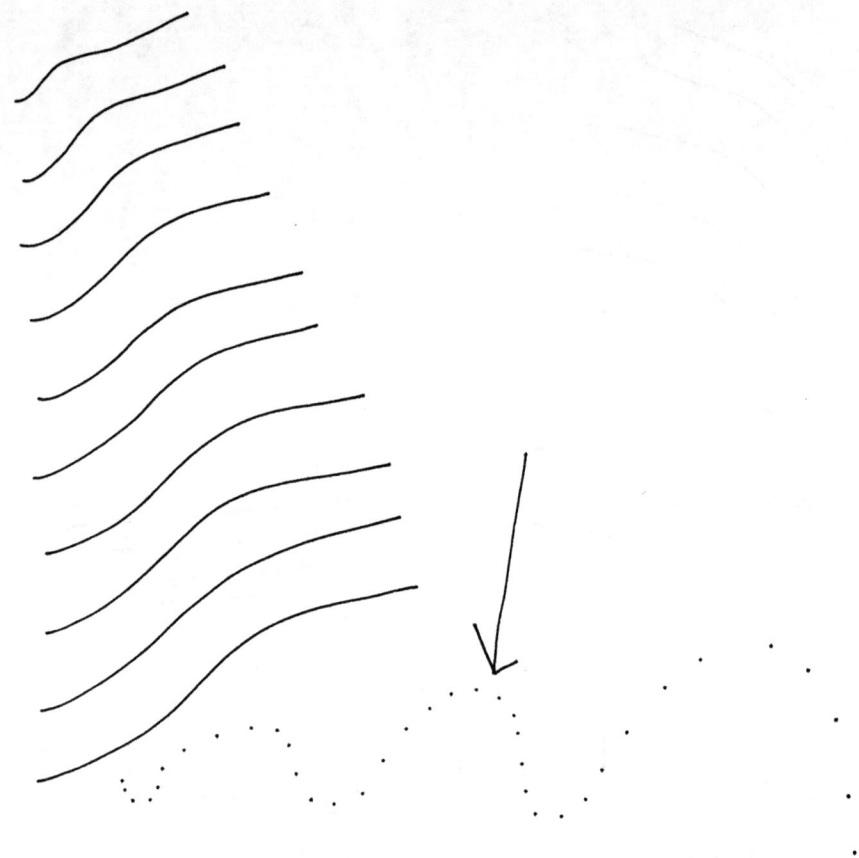

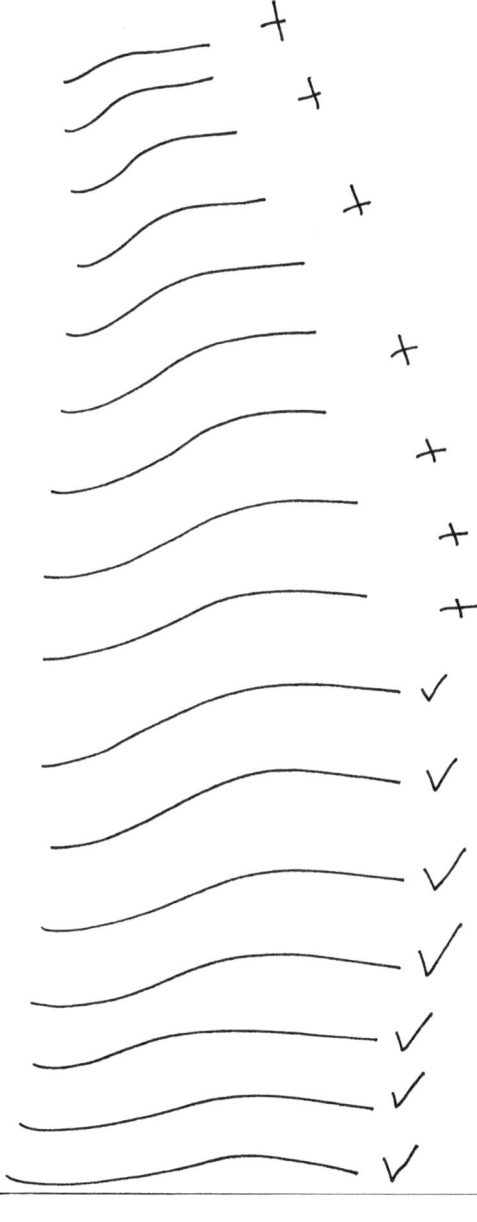

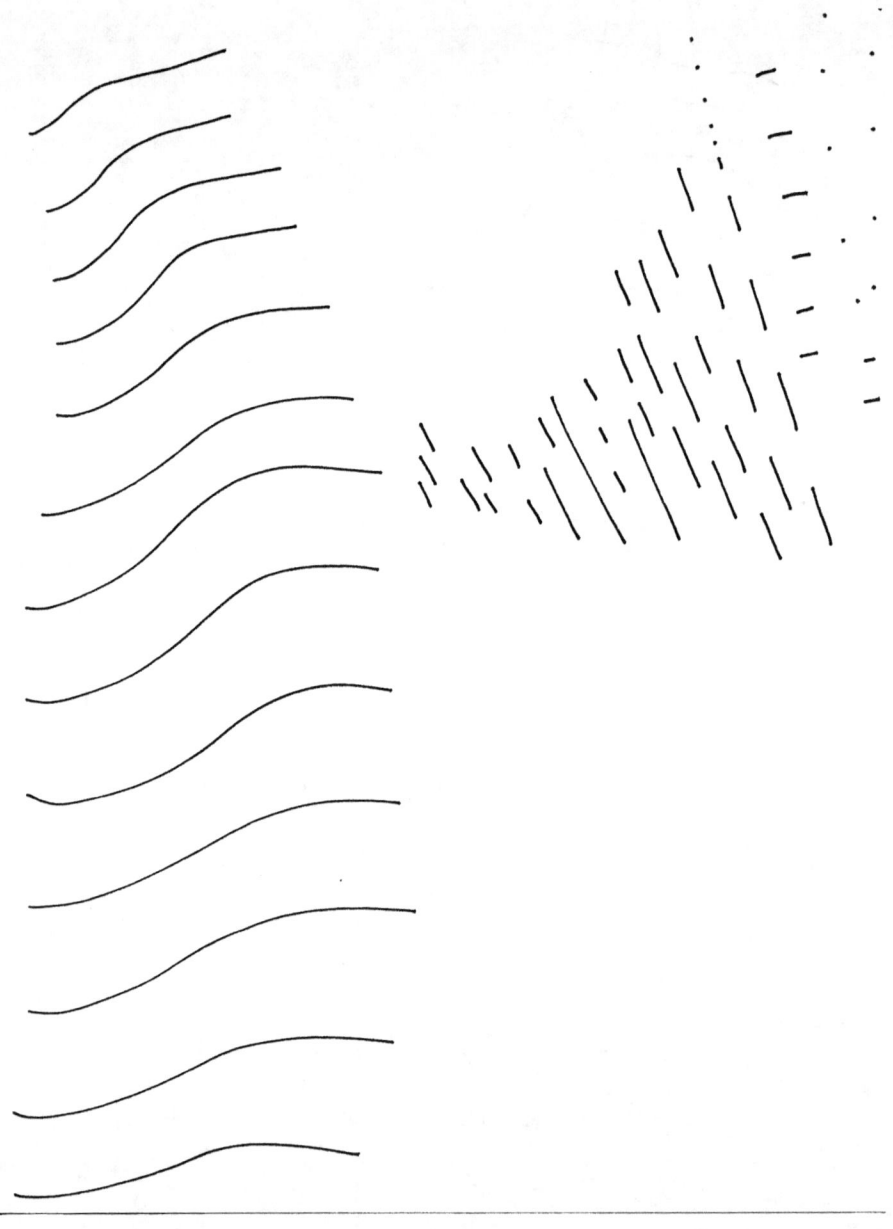

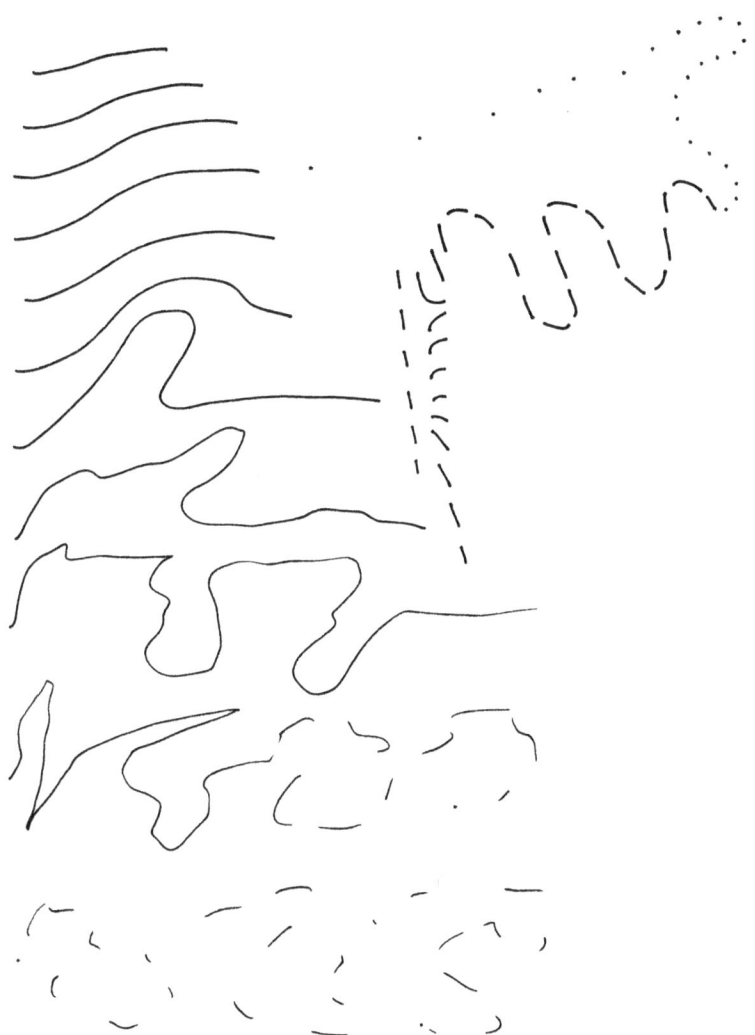

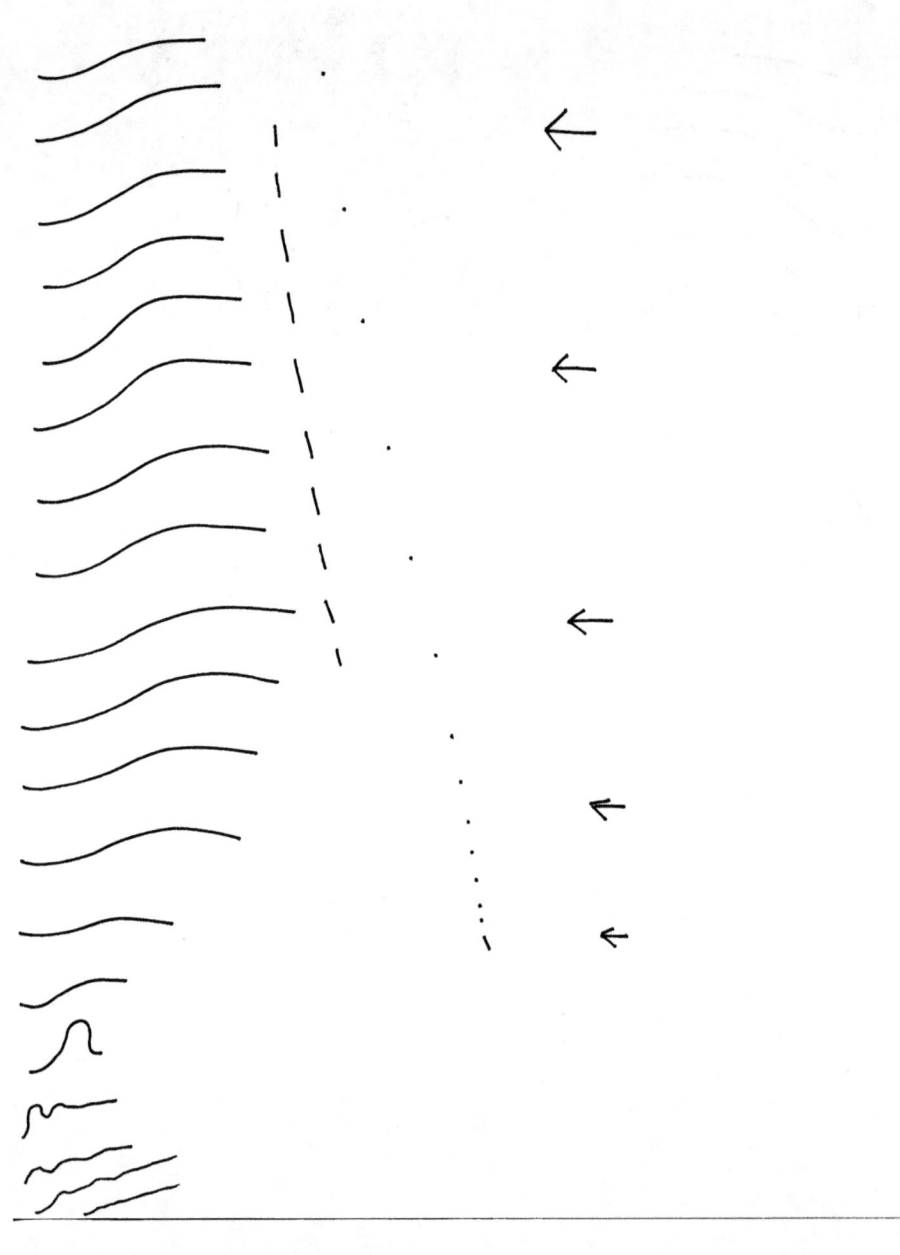

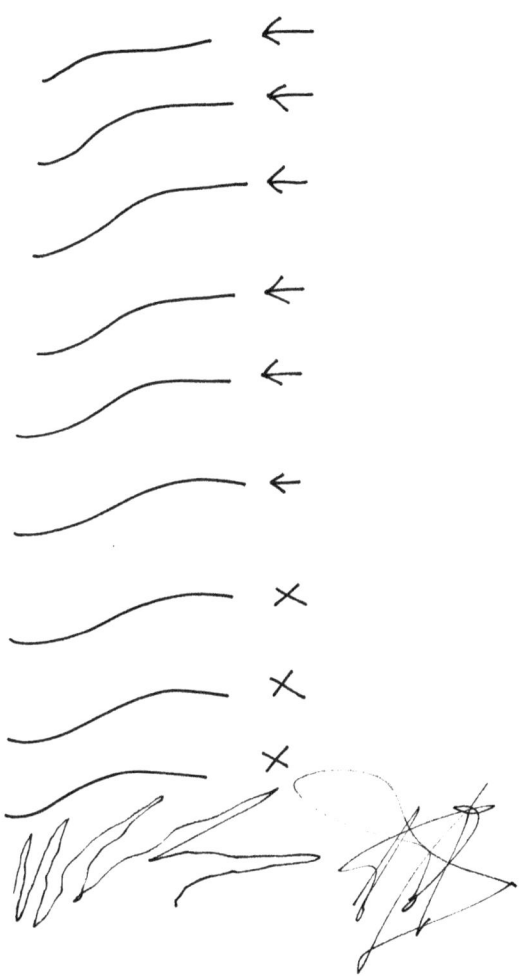

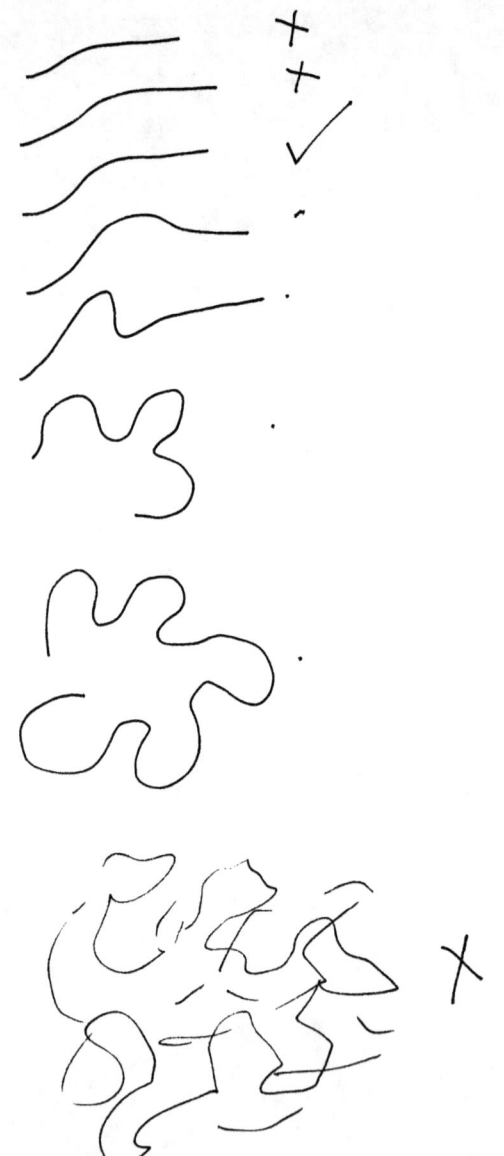

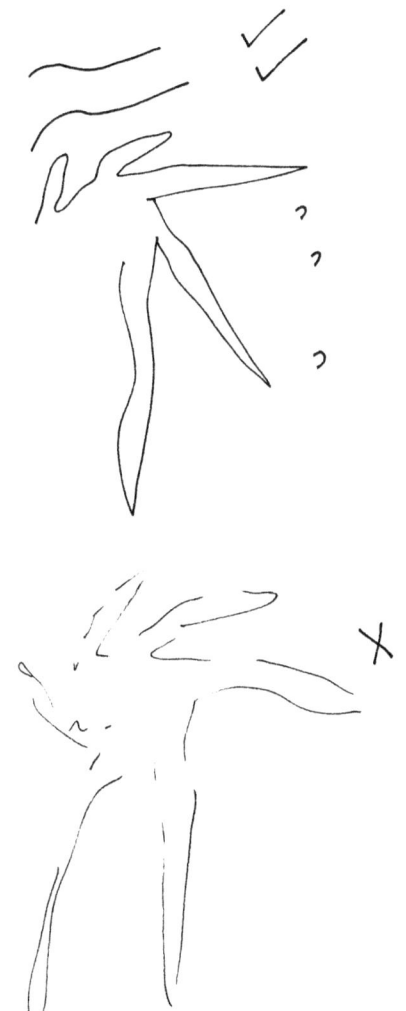

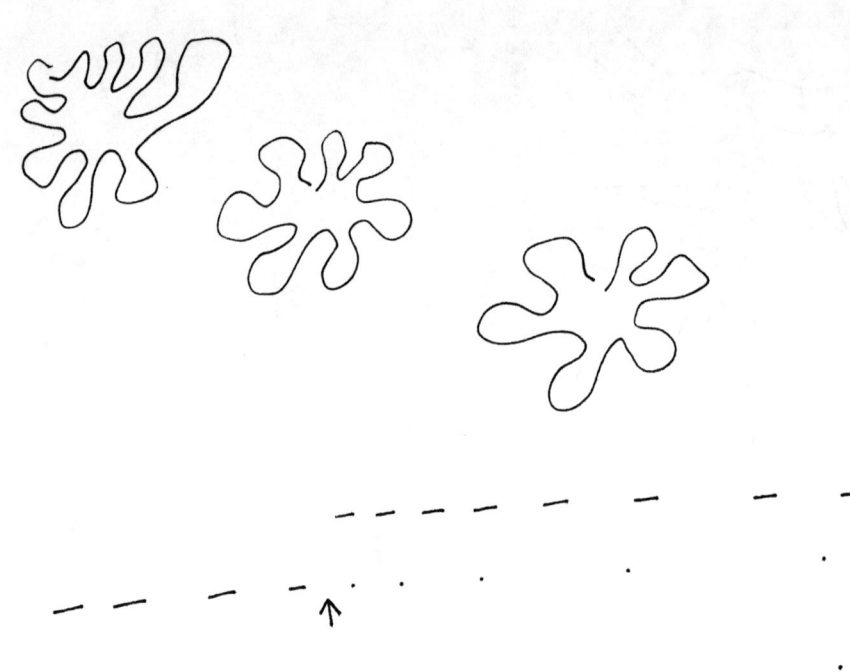

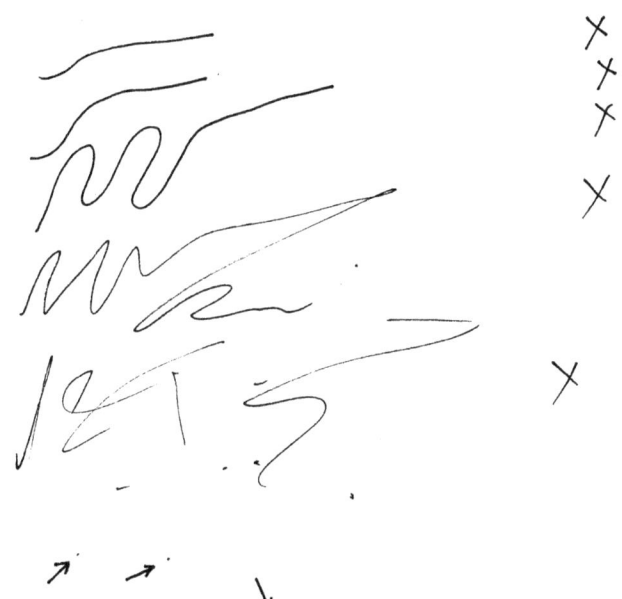

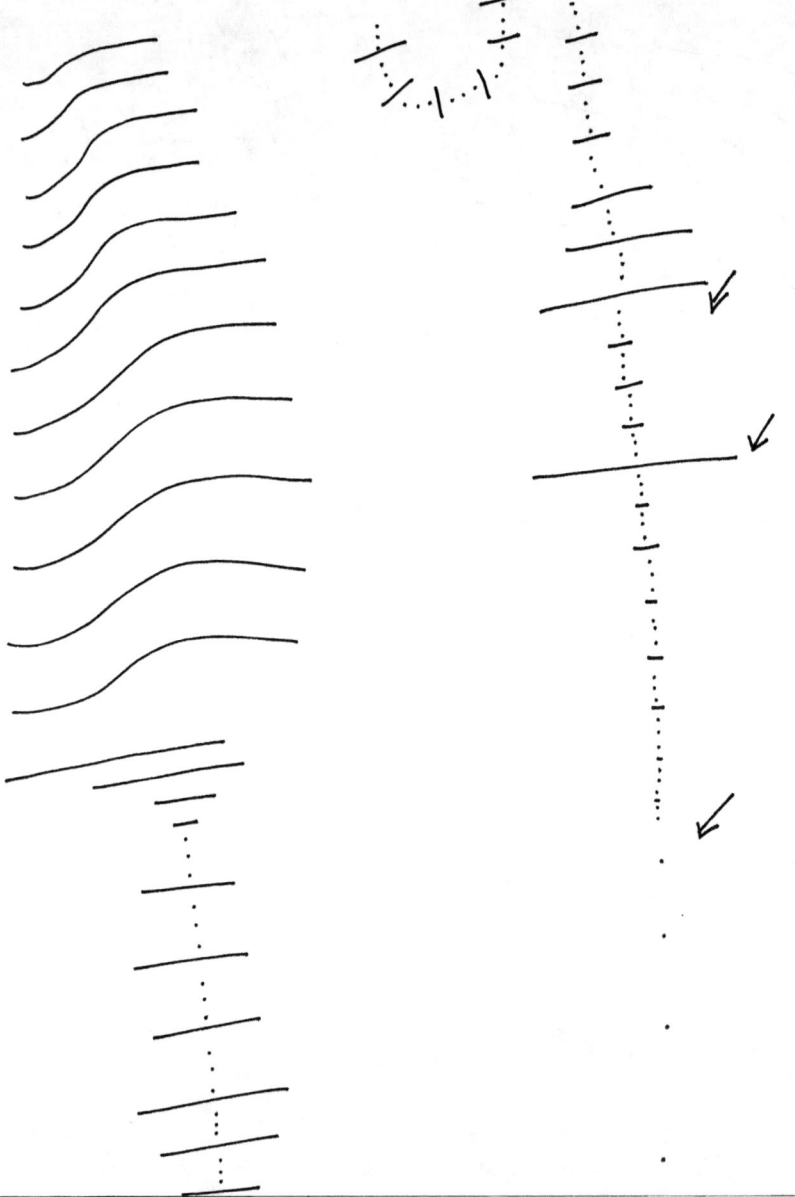

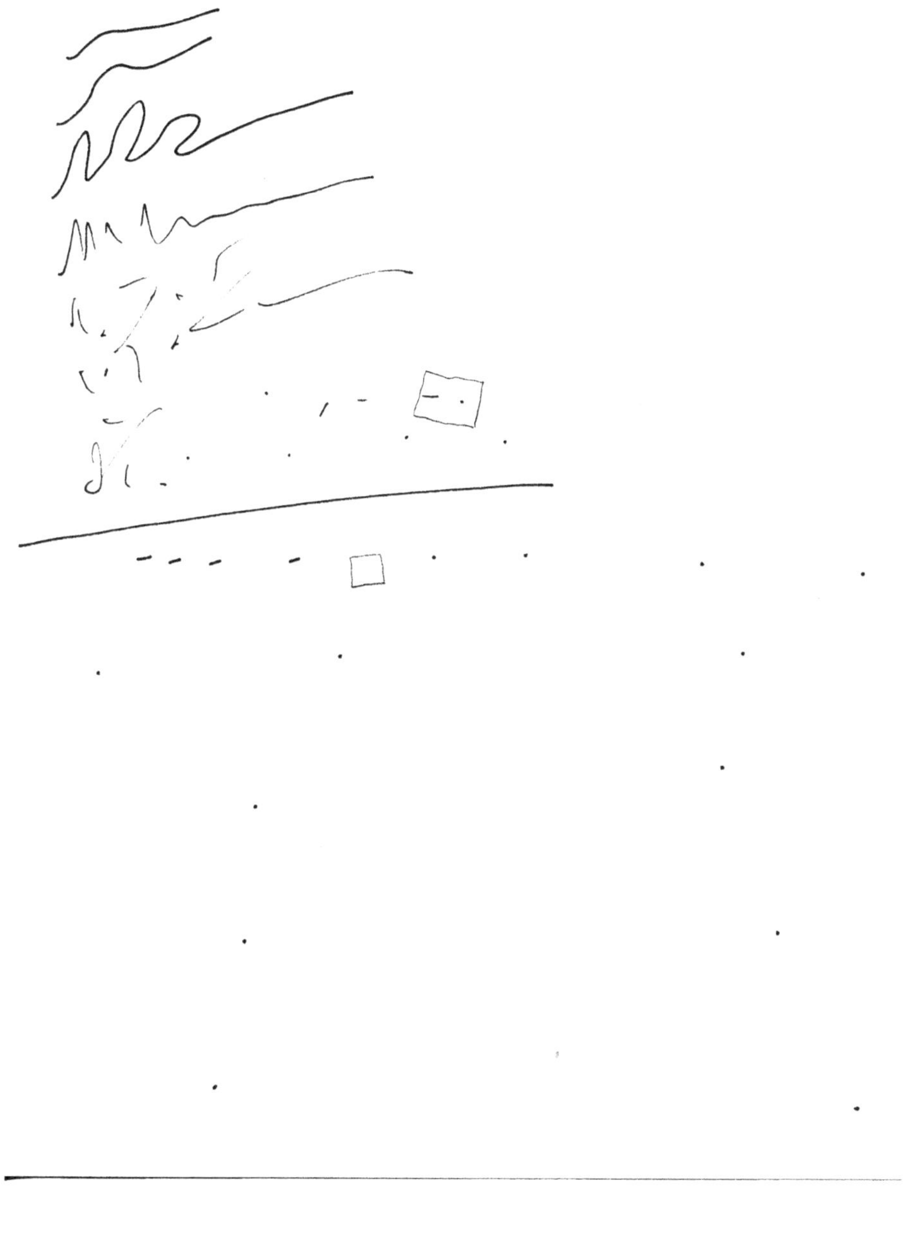

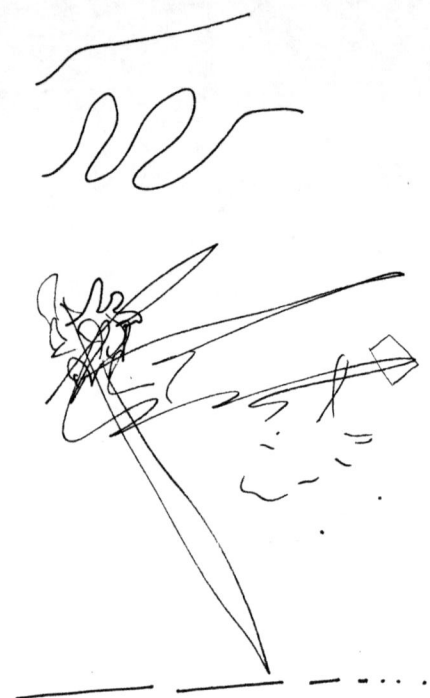

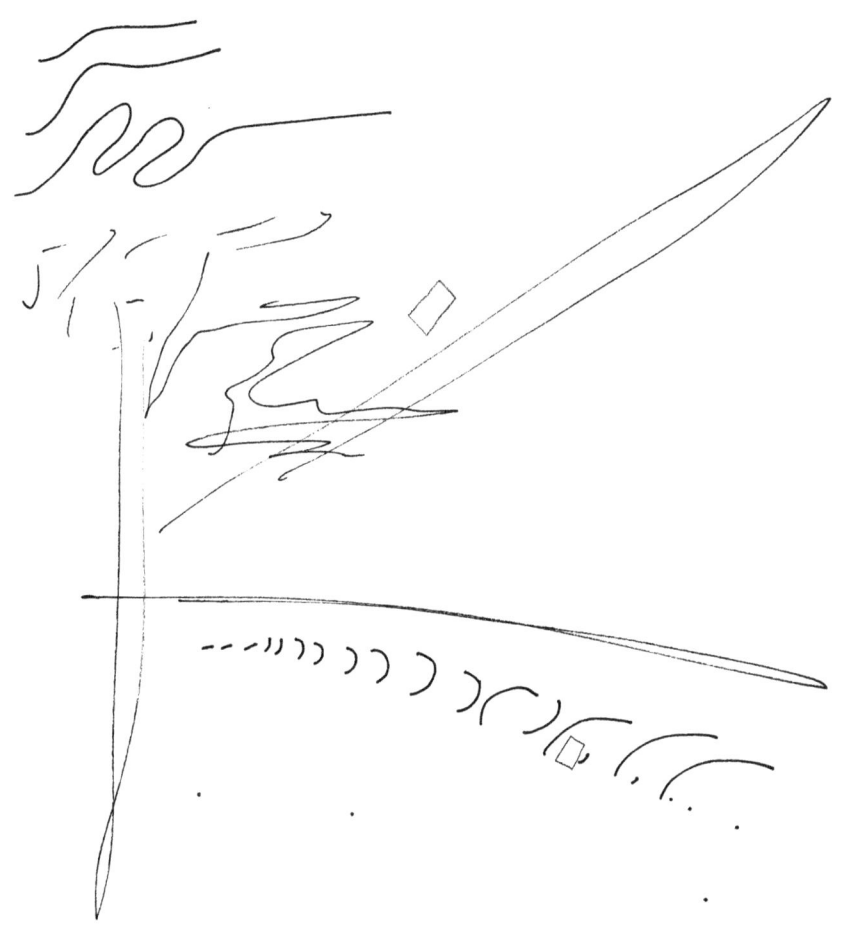

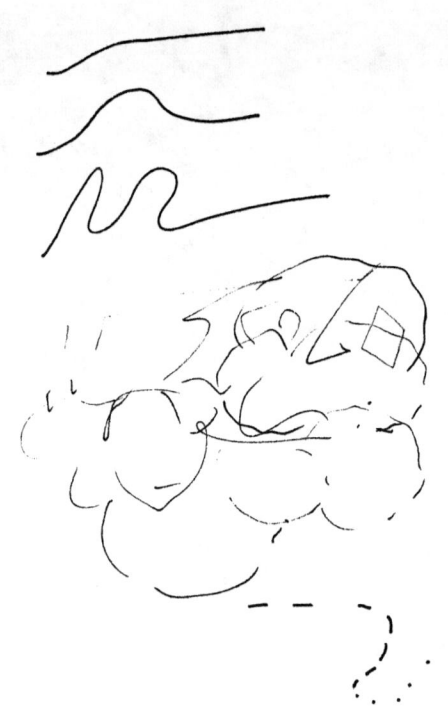

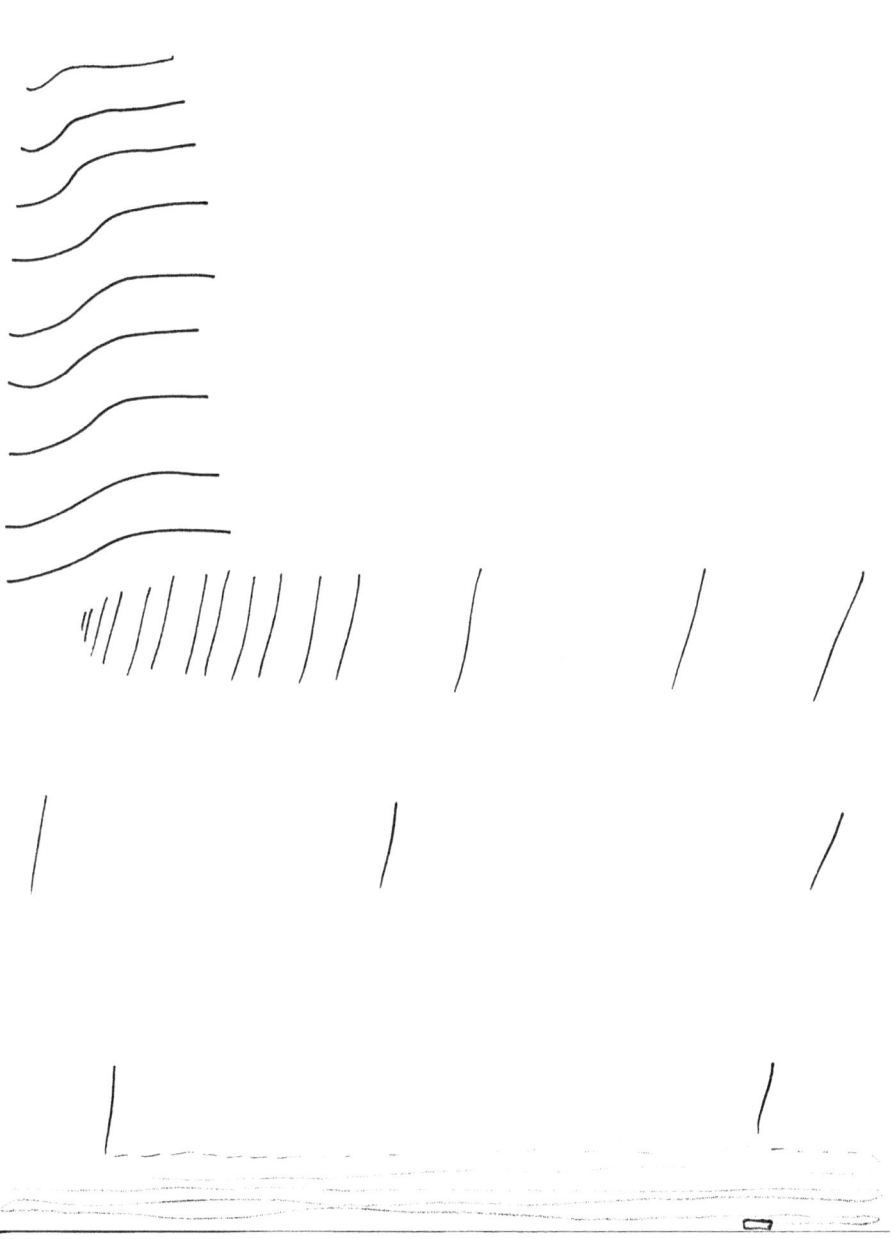

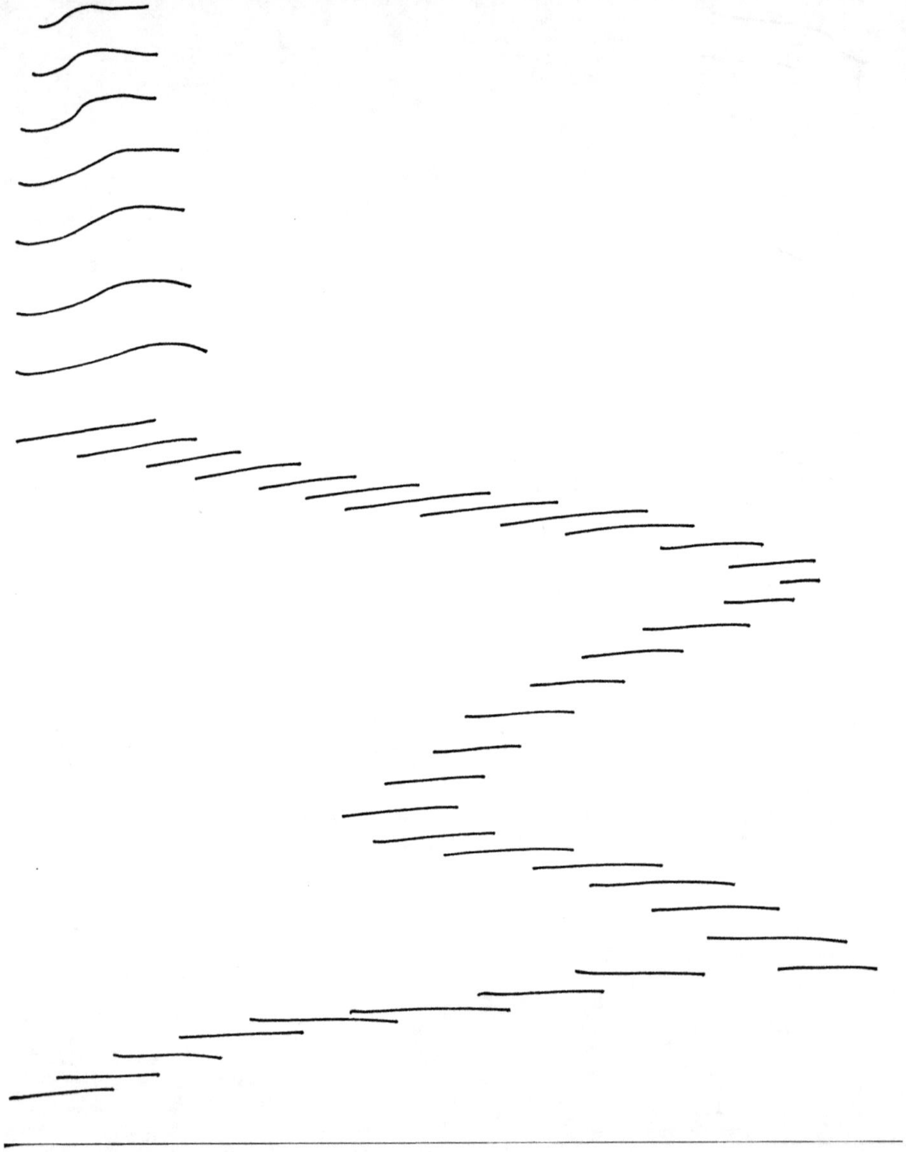